# Pharmacy Registration Assessment Questions


## Nadia Bukhari (Series Managing Editor)

BPharm (Hons), MRPharmS, PG Dip (Pharm Prac), PG Dip (T&L in Higher Ed), FHEA, FRPharmS
Senior Teaching Fellow, Pre-registration Co-ordinator, UCL School of Pharmacy, London, UK and Chairwoman, Pre-registration Conferences, Royal Pharmaceutical Society

## Oksana Pyzik (Assistant Editor and Contributor)

MRPharmS
Teaching Fellow, Department of Practice and Policy, UCL School of Pharmacy, London, UK

## Ryan Hamilton (Contributor)

MFRPSI, MRPharmS, MPharm (Hons), MIPharmM, AMRSC, AFHEA
Specialist Pharmacist in Antimicrobials, University Hospitals of Leicester NHS Trust

## Amar Iqbal (Contributor)

MPharm (Hons), MRPharmS, PG Dip (Clin Pharm)
Deputy Chief Pharmacist, Birmingham Women's Hospital, Pre-registration and Student Development Lead, RPS Birmingham and Solihull, and active member of the Neonatal and Paediatric Pharmacists Group

## Babir Malik (Contributor)

BSc (Hons), MRPharmS, PG Dip (Comm Pharm)
Pharmacist Manager for HI Weldricks Pharmacy and Pre-registration Lead for Sheffield, Rotherham and Barnsley Local Practice Forum




Pharmaceutical Press

**Published by the Pharmaceutical Press**
66–68 East Smithfield, London E1W 1AW, UK



Pharmaceutical Press is the publishing division of the Royal Pharmaceutical Society

First published 2016

Typeset by SPi Global, Chennai, India
Printed in Great Britain by Hobbs the Printers, Totton, Hampshire

ISBN 978 0 85711 175 3 (print)
ISBN 978 0 85711 266 8 (epdf)
ISBN 978 0 85711 267 5 (ePub)
ISBN 978 0 85711 268 2 (mobi)



A catalogue record for this book is available from the British Library

**Disclaimer**

**The views expressed in this book are solely those of the author and do not necessarily reflect the views or policies of the Royal Pharmaceutical Society. This book does NOT guarantee success in the registration exam but can be used as an aid for revision.**

I would like to dedicate this book to my children, Hamza and Myra Bukhari, who have given me the opportunity to be their role model.

# Contents

**Answers**

# Preface

After the overwhelming success of our first four volumes of *Registration Exam Questions*, a decision was made to launch a new series named *Pharmacy Registration Assessment Questions* (PRAQ). This new series hopes to incorporate questions that are aligned to the new GPhC Framework and incorporate a similar style of questions as recently announced by the GPhC for the Registration Assessment.

This book is a bank of just under 500 questions, which are similar to the style of the registration examination. The questions are based on law and ethics, and clinical pharmacy and therapeutic aspects of the registration examination syllabus, as well as pharmaceutical calculations.

After completing four years of study and graduating with a Master of Pharmacy (MPharm) degree, graduates are required to undertake training as a pre-registration pharmacist before they can sit the registration examination.

Pre-registration training is the period of employment on which graduates must embark and effectively complete before they can register as a pharmacist in the UK. In most cases it is a one-year period following the pharmacy degree; for sandwich course students it is integrated within the undergraduate programme.

On successfully passing the registration examination, pharmacy graduates can register as a pharmacist in the UK.

The registration examination harmonises the testing of skills in practice during the pre-registration year. It tests:

- knowledge
- the application of knowledge
- calculation
- time management
- managing stress
- comprehension
- recall
- interpretation
- evaluation

There are two examination papers: a closed book paper and a calculations paper. Questions are based on practice-based situations and are designed to test the thinking and knowledge that lie behind any action.

## EXAMINATION FORMAT

The registration examination consists of two papers:

1 calculation style

- free text answers; calculators can be used (provided by GPhC)
- 40 calculations in 120 minutes (2 hours)

2 closed book

- multiple-choice question (MCQ) paper with extracts from reference sources provided
- 120 questions in 150 minutes (2.5 hours)

Two types of MCQs are used:

- 90 best of five questions
- 30 extended matching questions

The registration examination is crucial for pharmacy graduates wishing to register in the UK.

Due to student demand, *Pharmacy Registration Assessment Questions* will be an annual publication with brand-new questions for students to attempt. We hope to include questions on most aspects of the examination and will take any changes made by the GPhC into consideration.

Preparation is the key. This book cannot guarantee that you will pass the registration examination; however, it can help you to practise the clinical pharmacy, pharmaceutical calculations, and law and ethics questions, all very important aspects of the registration examination, and, as they say, 'practice makes perfect'.

This book is written with the most current BNF at the time of writing. Please use the most current BNF and reference sources when using this book.

Good luck with the examination.

Nadia Bukhari
March 2016

# Acknowledgements

The editor wishes to acknowledge the support from colleagues at the UCL School of Pharmacy. Thank you to all four contributors – Ryan Hamilton, Oksana Pyzik, Amar Iqbal and Babir Malik.

Nadia Bukhari would like to express thanks to our editors at Pharmaceutical Press for their support and patience in the writing of this book, and especially to Christina Karaviotis and Vikarn Chowdhary for their guidance.

# About the authors

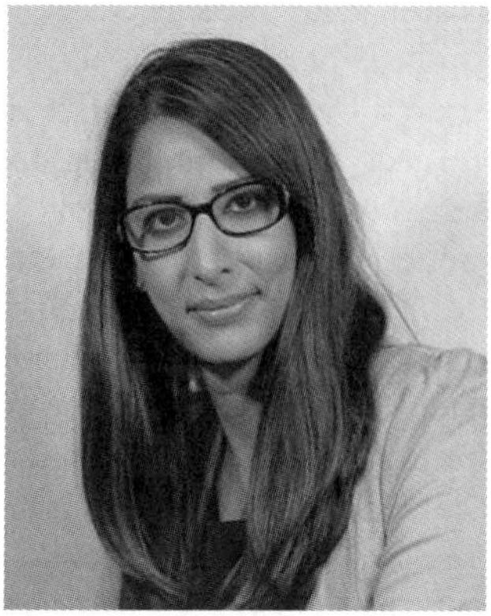

**Nadia Bukhari** is the Chair for the RPS Pre-registration Conferences. She developed the extremely popular and over-subscribed conference, when it first started in 2012. Nadia graduated from the School of Pharmacy, University of London in 1999. After qualifying, she worked as a pharmacy manager at Westbury Chemist, Streatham for a year, after which she moved on to work for Bart's and the London NHS Trust as a clinical pharmacist in surgery. It was at this time that Nadia developed an interest in teaching, as part of her role involved the responsibility of being a teacher practitioner for the School of Pharmacy, University of London. Two and a half years later, she commenced working for the School of Pharmacy, University of London as the pre-registration co-ordinator and the academic facilitator. This position involved teaching therapeutics to Master of Pharmacy students and assisting the director of undergraduate studies.

While teaching undergraduate students, Nadia completed her Post Graduate Diploma in Pharmacy Practice and her Post Graduate Diploma in Teaching in Higher Education. She then took on the role of the Master of Pharmacy Programme Manager, which involved the management of the undergraduate degree as well as being the pre-registration co-ordinator for the university.

Since the merger with UCL, Nadia has now taken on the role of Senior Teaching Fellow in Pharmacy Practice and is the pre-registration co-ordinator for the university. She is also a Fellow of the Higher Education Academy. Nadia has recently taken on the responsibility of course co-ordinator for the final year of the MPharm.

Taking her research interest further, Nadia is currently in the third year of her PhD, which she is doing on a part-time basis. Her research area is 'Professional Leadership in Pharmacy'.

Nadia's interest in writing emerged in her first year of working in academia. Thirteen years on, Nadia has authored six titles with the Pharmaceutical Press. She is currently writing her seventh title, which is due to be published in February 2017.

Nadia has recently been awarded the status of Fellow of the Royal Pharmaceutical Society, for her distinction in the Profession of Pharmacy.

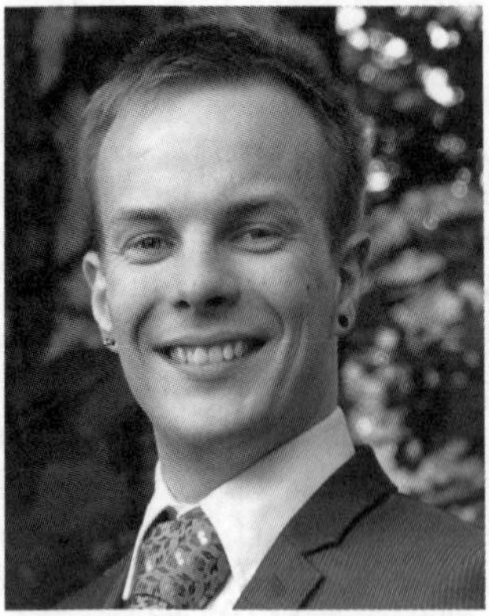

**Ryan Hamilton** is a specialist pharmacist at University Hospitals of Leicester NHS Trust where he works within the fields of antimicrobials and acute medicine.

Ryan studied pharmacy at Liverpool John Moores University (LJMU) to which he returned, after completing his pre-registration training at King's College Hospital, to undertake a PhD in pharmaceutical sciences. His research is investigating the interaction of antimicrobial agents with clay minerals and the development of candidate materials, containing these novel clay mineral complexes, for the treatment of infected wounds. During his time as a PhD candidate at LJMU, Ryan taught on a number of key components of the pharmacy degree, eventually being awarded associate fellowship of the Higher Education Academy.

Throughout his career Ryan has supported pharmacy students and pre-registration pharmacists. As President of the British Pharmaceutical Students' Association, he developed guidance for students and trainees, and worked closely with the GPhC to ensure trainees were fairly represented. Ryan now acts as an ambassador for the BPSA and sits on the RPS's Education Forum where he represents trainees and foundation year pharmacists. He is also an active member of the UK Clinical Pharmacy Association where he regularly adjudicates abstracts for the Association's symposia, and previously sat on the General Committee.

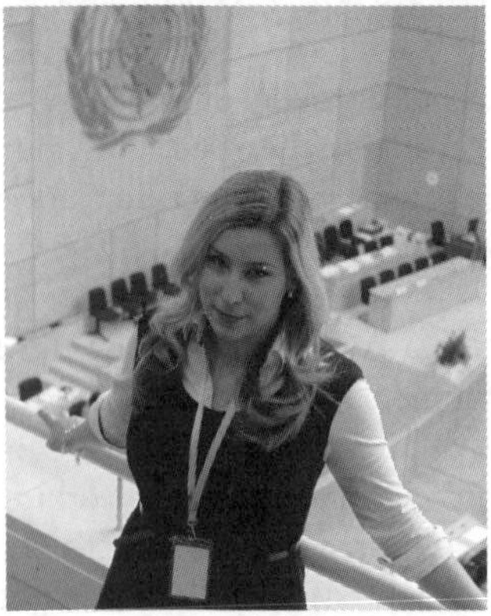

**Oksana Pyzik** is a Teaching Fellow at the UCL School of Pharmacy in the Department of Practice and Policy. She is a current member of the Royal Pharmaceutical Society (RPS) Pre-registration Advisory Group and is the Pre-registration and Academic Lead alongside Nadia Bukhari for the Central London Local Practice Forum (LPF). Oksana is extensively involved with the Royal Pharmaceutical Society (RPS) Pre-registration Conferences in the development of teaching material as well as delivering the training sessions as part of the RPS Pre-registration Teaching Panel.

Oksana first started her career as a pharmacist in the primary care setting delivering public health interventions to marginalised patient groups in underserved communities across London. It was this early experience in practice that motivated her to conduct public health research at the International Pharmaceutical Federation in The Hague, before switching into the academic sector full time in 2013. She went on to earn her Post Graduate Diploma in Teaching and Learning in Higher Professional Education at the Institute of Education in 2015 and is now a Fellow of the UK Higher Education Academy.

Her research interests also expand outside pharmacy education and professionalism to include public health and policy, and global health. She was selected as the UCL Global Citizenship Programme Leader on Ebola due to run in June 2016 and is part of the Global Pharmacist Initiative. Oksana is the current Academic Lead of the UCL Fight the Fakes Campaign against Counterfeit Medicines and was also partnered with the United Nations Secretary General's Envoy on Youth to review the 'Global Partnership for Youth in the Post 2015 Development Agenda' for the UN Economic and Social Council Youth Forum in 2014. In addition to her teaching and research, Oksana provides pastoral care for international students as the International Student Advisor at the UCL School of Pharmacy and is an education consultant for the International Study Centre at the University of Surrey.

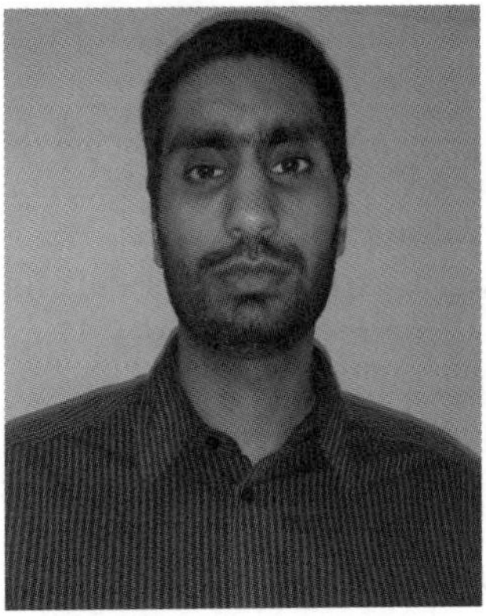

**Amar Iqbal** graduated with first-class honours from Aston University in 2007 and completed his pre-registration year with Alliance Boots in a busy community pharmacy in Warwickshire. Amar's skills were quickly recognised and upon qualification in 2008 he went on to become store manager at the UK's first ever hospital outpatient pharmacy collaboration. Amar switched to the NHS in 2010 while also completing his Post Graduate Clinical Diploma a year later. It was here he gained a broad experience of medical and surgical wards, emergency admissions and medicines information among other things while at Sandwell and West Birmingham Hospitals NHS Trust. Following this, Amar specialised in neonatal intensive care, paediatrics, surgical day-case and maternity ward areas while serving as a Senior Clinical Pharmacist and Teacher Practitioner at the Heart of England NHS Foundation Teaching Trust. Here he was involved in policy and formulary writing, reviewing financial reports, as well as being closely involved in inducting, training and educating healthcare professionals. This included working on an in-house prescribing module (VITAL) as well as working with the local medical deanery on a paediatric SCRIPT prescribing module. Amar's role with Aston University involved working with students on patient-centred learning within the hospital setting, as well as workshops and clinical assessments at university. Amar went on to work as an Independent Pharmaceutical Consultant and locum pharmacist. Currently, Amar is enjoying his role as Deputy Chief Pharmacist at Birmingham Women's Hospital.

Amar is a keen advocate of the Royal Pharmaceutical Society (RPS) and has a dedicated role as Pre-registration and Student Development Lead at multi-award winning Birmingham and Solihull Local Practice Forum. He also sits on the RPS Pre-registration Advisory Panel helping to provide support material for upcoming pharmacists. In addition to this, Amar has reviewed national guidance, had valuable input into local and national pharmacy initiatives, and has worked for both the RPSGB and now GPhC.

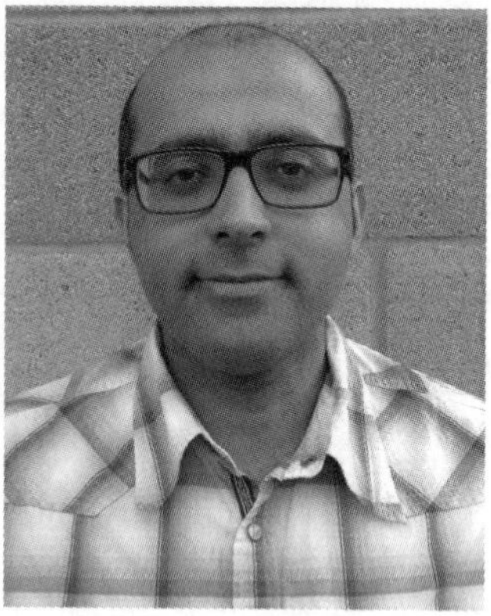

**Babir Malik** graduated from Bradford University in 2007 after doing consecutive degrees in Biomedical Sciences and Pharmacy. He did his pre-registration training at Weldricks Pharmacy in Rotherham and now works at Weldricks Pharmacy in Scunthorpe. He did his Post Graduate Diploma in Community Pharmacy at Keele University.

Babir is a former pre-registration tutor and has also sat on the Rotherham Local Pharmaceutical Committee. He is currently the Pre-registration Lead for Sheffield, Rotherham and Barnsley Local Practice Forum.

Babir is a Dementia Friends Champion and has made over 300 Dementia Friends. He is passionate about working with pharmacy students and pre-registration trainee pharmacists and is on the RPS Pre-registration Panel for their revision conferences.

# Abbreviations

| | |
|---|---|
| ACBS | Advisory Committee on Borderline Substances |
| ACE | angiotensin-converting enzyme |
| ACEI | angiotensin-converting enzyme inhibitor |
| ALT DIE | alternate days |
| AV | arteriovenous |
| BD | twice daily |
| BMI | body mass index |
| BNF | *British National Formulary* |
| BNFC | *British National Formulary for Children* |
| BP | blood pressure |
| bpm | beats per minute |
| BPSA | British Pharmaceutical Students' Association |
| BSA | body surface area |
| BTS | British Thoracic Society |
| CCF | congestive/chronic cardiac failure |
| CD | controlled drug |
| CE | *conformité européenne* |
| CFC | chlorofluorocarbon |
| CHM | Commission on Human Medicines |
| CHMP | Committee for Medicinal Products for Human Use |
| COX | cyclooxygenase |
| COPD | chronic obstructive pulmonary disease |
| CPD | continuing professional development |
| CPPE | Centre for Pharmacy Postgraduate Education |
| CrCl | creatinine clearance (mL/minute) |
| CSM | Committee on Safety of Medicines |
| CYT | cytochrome |
| DigCl | digoxin clearance (L/hour) |
| DMARD | disease-modifying antirheumatic drug |
| DNG | discount not given |
| DPF | *Dental Practitioners' Formulary* |
| EC | enteric-coated |
| ECG | electrocardiogram |
| EEA | European Economic Area |

| | |
|---|---|
| eGFR | estimated glomerular filtration rate |
| EHC | emergency hormonal contraception |
| F1 | Foundation Year 1 |
| $FEV_1$ | forced expiratory volume in 1 second |
| GP | general practitioner |
| GP6D | glucose-6-phosphate dehydrogenase |
| GPhC | General Pharmaceutical Council |
| GSL | general sales list |
| GTN | glyceryl trinitrate |
| HbA1c | glycated haemoglobin |
| HDU | high dependency unit |
| HIV | human immunodeficiency virus |
| HR | heart rate |
| HRT | hormone replacement therapy |
| IBS | irritable bowel syndrome |
| IBW | ideal body weight |
| IDA | industrial denatured alcohol |
| IM | intramuscular |
| INR | international normalised ratio |
| IV | intravenous |
| IUD | intrauterine device |
| MAOI | monoamine oxidase inhibitor |
| MD | maximum single dose |
| MDD | maximum daily dose |
| MDI | metered-dose inhaler |
| MDU | to be used as directed |
| MEP | *Medicines, Ethics and Practice* guide |
| MHRA | Medicines and Healthcare products Regulatory Agency |
| MMR | measles, mumps and rubella |
| MR, m/r | modified release |
| MUPS | multiple-unit pellet system |
| MUR | Medicines Use Review |
| NHS | National Health Service |
| NICE | National Institute for Health and Care Excellence |
| NMS | New Medicines Service |
| NRLS | National Reporting and Learning System |
| NSAIDs | non-steroidal anti-inflammatory drugs |
| OC | oral contraceptive |
| OD | omni die (every day) |
| OM | omni mane (every morning) |

| | |
|---|---|
| ON | omni nocte (every night) |
| OP | original pack |
| OPAT | outpatient parenteral antibacterial therapy |
| ORT | oral rehydration therapy |
| OTC | over-the-counter |
| P | pharmacy |
| PAGB | Proprietary Association of Great Britain |
| PCT | primary care trust |
| PIL | patient information leaflet |
| PMH | past medical history |
| PMR | patient medical record |
| POM | prescription-only medicine |
| POM-V | prescription-only medicine – veterinarian |
| POM-VPS | prescription-only medicine – veterinarian, pharmacist, suitably qualified person |
| PPIs | proton pump inhibitors |
| PRN | when required |
| PSA | prostate-specific antigen |
| PSNC | Pharmaceutical Services Negotiating Committee |
| QDS | quarter die sumendum (to be taken four times daily) |
| RE | right eye |
| RPS | Royal Pharmaceutical Society (formerly RPSGB) |
| SARSS | Suspected Adverse Reaction Surveillance Scheme |
| SCRIPT | Standard Computerised Revalidation Instrument for Prescribing and Therapeutics |
| SeCr | serum creatinine |
| SHO | senior house officer |
| SIGN | Scottish Intercollegiate Guidelines Network |
| SLS | selected list scheme |
| SOP | standard operating procedure |
| SPC | summary of product characteristics |
| SSRI | selective serotonin reuptake inhibitor |
| ST | an isoelectric line after the QRS complex of an ECG |
| STAT | immediately |
| TCA | tricyclic antidepressant |
| TDS | three times a day |
| TPN | total parenteral nutrition |
| TSDA | trade-specific denatured alcohol |
| U&E | urea and electrolyte count |
| UTI | urinary tract infection |
| VITAL | Virtual Interactive Teaching And Learning |
| WHO | World Health Organization |

# Changes to the assessment

*Taken from the GPhC website*:

The changes which the board of assessors have agreed are:

- Replacing all open book source references, including the BNF, with artefacts from clinical practice, such as patient information leaflets, which candidates will need to use to answer questions
- Allowing calculators to be used in one of the papers
- Removing multiple completion and assertion reason questions, and introducing a new type of MCQ, so that there are two types of questions – best of five and extended matching questions
- Reformatting the assessment syllabus so that it is mapped to the current Future Pharmacists learning outcomes, and to make sure that the assessment covers the appropriate areas of the learning outcomes

For more information, please visit:

https://www.pharmacyregulation.org/2016_changes

# How to use this book

The book is divided into three main sections: best of five questions, extended matching questions and calculation questions.

## BEST OF FIVE QUESTIONS

Each of the questions or statements in this section is followed by five suggested answers. Select the best answer in each situation.

For example:
A patient on your ward has been admitted with a gastric ulcer, which is currently being treated. She has a history of arthritis and cardiac problems. Which of her drugs is most likely to have caused the gastric ulcer?

☐ A paracetamol
☐ B naproxen
☐ C furosemide
☐ D propranolol
☐ E codeine phosphate

## EXTENDED MATCHING QUESTIONS

Extended matching questions consist of lettered options followed by a list of numbered problems/questions. For each numbered problem/question select the one lettered option that most closely answers the question. You can use the lettered options once, more than once, or not at all.

For example:

**Antibacterials**

A ciprofloxacin
B co-amoxiclav
C co-trimoxazole
D doxycycline
E erythromycin
F flucloxacillin
G metronidazole
H nitrofurantoin

For the patient described, select the single most likely antibacterial agent from the list above. Each option may be used once, more than once or not at all.
Mr S comes into your pharmacy with a prescription for a short course of an antibacterial after a dental procedure. You advise the patient to avoid alcohol and that he may experience taste disturbance and furred tongue.

## CALCULATION QUESTIONS

The GPhC will expect candidates to bring in their own calculator for the purpose of the assessment. Models they will allow are the Aurora HC133, Aurora DT210, or Casio MX8-S.

For example:
Miss Q has been admitted to hospital and is undergoing cardiac surgery. She has received a continuous infusion of dobutamine for the procedure and the infusion device was set 10 hours ago. The patient weighs 50 kg and the infusion device was set at 5 mcg/kg per minute. Calculate the amount of dobutamine (mg) that a patient has received while on a continuous infusion.

The purpose of the registration assessment is to test a candidate's ability to apply the knowledge they have learnt throughout the previous five years of their education and training.

Testing someone's ability to locate information efficiently in the BNF should be tested during their pre-registration training year and in their undergraduate training. Therefore, all questions are closed book, with extracts of reference sources provided to candidates.

Answers to the questions are at the end of the book. Brief explanations or a suitable reference for sourcing the answer are given to aid understanding and to facilitate learning.

Important: this text refers to the edition of the BNF current when the text was written. Please always consult the LATEST version for the most up-to-date information.

# *Best of five questions*

## SECTION A

Ryan Hamilton

Questions 1–3 concern Mrs G who is a patient on your respiratory ward. Upon clinically screening her drug chart you determine she is on the following:

Salbutamol 100 mcg/actuation CFC-free inhaler, 2–6 puffs PRN
Tiotropium 18 mcg OM
*Symbicort* 400/12 *Turbohaler* one puff BD
Paracetamol 500–1000 mg QDS PRN
Prednisolone 30 mg OM 10/7
Doxycycline 200 mg OM 10/7

1 Mrs G has developed a sore mouth over the past 24 hours. On examination the inside of her cheeks and tongue look red and raw and the doctor asks for your opinion. You suspect the newly started *Symbicort* may have precipitated this condition.
Which of the following would be the most appropriate initial treatment for Mrs G?

☐ A co-amoxiclav 625 mg TDS
☐ B *Difflam* (benzydamine hydrochloride) 15 mL QDS
☐ C fluconazole 50 mg OD
☐ D itraconazole 100 mg BD
☐ E nystatin (100 000 units/mL) 1 mL QDS

2 You decide to talk to Mrs G about her inhalers and counsel her on the best inhaler technique.
Which of the following instructions would you give regarding *Symbicort*?

☐ A Inhale quickly and deeply
☐ B Inhale quickly and shallowly
☐ C Inhale slowly and deeply
☐ D Inhale slowly and gently
☐ E Offer Mrs G a spacer

3 Mrs G asks how she can avoid developing a sore mouth in the future. Which of the following would you advise when using *Symbicort*?

☐ A Hold breath for 10 seconds
☐ B Only use when wheezy
☐ C Rinse mouth after use
☐ D Use a spacer
☐ E None of the above; the condition cannot be prevented

4 You are reviewing the medicines for a patient newly admitted to your stroke unit, Mr W. Due to impaired swallow he has had a nasogastric tube inserted.
Which of the following medicines should not be crushed or dispersed to go down the tube?

☐ A *Chemydur 60XL* (isosorbide mononitrate)
☐ B clopidogrel 75 mg tablets
☐ C paracetamol 500 mg dispersible tablets
☐ D ramipril 2.5 mg capsules
☐ E simvastatin 40 mg tablets

Questions 5–7 concern Mr F who is one of your regular mental health patients who has come to collect his clozapine. Mr F's mental health specialist is currently prescribing clozapine 100 mg in the morning, 100 mg in the afternoon and 150 mg in the evening.
Using the summary of product characteristics via the following link answer the questions that follow: http://www.medicines.org.uk/emc/medicine/1277.

5 Before dispensing the clozapine you decide to check Mr F's blood results.
Which of the following levels do you need to ensure are in range?

- ☐ A phosphate levels
- ☐ B potassium levels
- ☐ C red blood cell count
- ☐ D sodium levels
- ☐ E white cell count

6 During your consultation with Mr F you discuss his recent admission to the local A&E department after falling on a night out.
Which of the following would be most appropriate to tell Mr F in relation to drinking alcohol?

- ☐ A It may make clozapine more effective
- ☐ B It may make clozapine less effective
- ☐ C It may increase likelihood of drowsiness
- ☐ D It may make Mr F more alert
- ☐ E Mr F should not drink while taking clozapine

7 Upon discussing his recent admission to hospital you learn that he has not taken his clozapine for around 3 days.
Which of these would be the most appropriate action to take?

- ☐ A Dispense the clozapine. Tell Mr F to take his normal dose and report any side-effects
- ☐ B Dispense the clozapine. Tell Mr F to take his normal dose and arrange to see specialist
- ☐ C Dispense the clozapine. Tell Mr F to take 12.5 mg today then return to his normal dose
- ☐ D Do not dispense the clozapine. Contact the specialist to discuss re-initiation
- ☐ E Do not dispense the clozapine. Send the patient back to hospital for re-initiation

Questions 8–10 concern Mr V has, who just been diagnosed with *Clostridium difficile* for the first time. You look at his drug chart and see the following:

| **Name:** Mr V **DOB:** 25/08/1958 **NHS No.:** 00 123 456 789 | | | | **Allergies and Reactions** *NKDA* | | | |
|---|---|---|---|---|---|---|---|
| **Weight:** 78 kg | | **Height:** | | | | | |
| Date 4/2/16 | Drug Cefuroxime | Dose 250 mg | Route PO | Date 4/2/16 | Drug Prednisolone | Dose 7.5 mg | Route PO |
| Indication ? LRTI | 08:00 / 12:00 | | | Indication Long term | 08:00 / 12:00 | | |
| Prescriber *Dr Smith* | 17:00 / 22:00 | | | Prescriber *Dr Smith* | 17:00 / 22:00 | | |
| Date 5/2/16 | Drug Candesartan | Dose 8 mg | Route PO | Date 5/2/16 | Drug Lactulose | Dose 10 ml | Route PO |
| Indication | 08:00 / 12:00 | | | Indication | 08:00 / 12:00 | | |
| Prescriber *Dr Patel* | 17:00 / 22:00 | | | Prescriber *Dr Patel* | 17:00 / 22:00 | | |
| Date 5/2/16 | Drug Aspirin | Dose 75 mg | Route PO | Date 5/2/16 | Drug Adcal D3 | Dose † | Route PO |
| Indication | 08:00 / 12:00 | | | Indication | 08:00 / 12:00 | | |
| Prescriber *Dr Patel* | 17:00 / 22:00 | | | Prescriber *Dr Patel* | 17:00 / 22:00 | | |
| Date 5/2/16 | Drug Lansoprazole | Dose 30 mg | Route PO | Date | Drug | Dose | Route |
| Indication | 08:00 / 12:00 | | | Indication | 08:00 / 12:00 | | |
| Prescriber *Dr Patel* | 17:00 / 22:00 | | | Prescriber | 17:00 / 22:00 | | |

8   Which of the following would be the most appropriate first-line treatment?

    ☐ **A**   fidaxomicin 200 mg BD PO
    ☐ **B**   metronidazole 400 mg TDS PO
    ☐ **C**   metronidazole 500 mg TDS IV
    ☐ **D**   vancomycin 125 mg QDS PO
    ☐ **E**   vancomycin 500 mg BD IV

9   Which of Mr V's concurrent medications may have precipitated the *C. difficile* infection?

    ☐ **A**   aspirin 75 mg OM
    ☐ **B**   candesartan 8 mg OM
    ☐ **C**   cefuroxime 250 mg BD
    ☐ **D**   lactulose 10 mL BD
    ☐ **E**   prednisolone 7.5 mg OM

**10** Which other of Mr V's medicines would you also withhold and review in relation to the *C. difficile* infection?

- ☐ A Adcal D3 one tablet BD
- ☐ B candesartan 8 mg OM
- ☐ C lansoprazole 30 mg OM
- ☐ D paracetamol 500 mg QDS PRN
- ☐ E prednisolone 7.5 mg OM

**11** Miss C has been prescribed doxycycline capsules 200 mg once daily for 5 days to treat a suspected lower respiratory tract infection.
When you are handing out this medicine, which of the following counselling points would you not need to tell her?

- ☐ A Avoid drinking milk and eating dairy close to doxycycline dose
- ☐ B Do not take indigestion remedies close to doxycycline dose
- ☐ C Do not use sunbeds while taking doxycycline
- ☐ D Take doxycycline with a full glass of water
- ☐ E Take doxycycline on an empty stomach

**12** Mr R has brought in a prescription to your community pharmacy for bumetanide 2 mg BD. Upon looking at his PMR you notice he has been taking bumetanide 2 mg OM for the past 6 months.
Which of the following courses of action would be the most appropriate?

- ☐ A Ask Mr R to go back to his GP to get a new prescription
- ☐ B Contact the prescriber as bumetanide should be given only once daily
- ☐ C Contact the prescriber as this is a likely prescribing error
- ☐ D Dispense the bumetanide, counselling Mr R to take the doses at 8 am and 2 pm
- ☐ E Dispense the bumetanide, counselling Mr R to take the doses at 8 am and 8 pm

**13** Mr N comes to your community pharmacy for an emergency supply of flecainide tablets, which he regularly takes. He ran out of his tablets last night and will not be able to get a prescription for at least 48 hours. You dispense the emergency supply to him and label the product.
Which of the following is not a requirement for the emergency supply dispensed label?

- ☐ **A** The address of your pharmacy
- ☐ **B** The date of dispensing
- ☐ **C** The name of the patient's GP
- ☐ **D** The total quantity of tablets dispensed
- ☐ **E** The words 'emergency supply'

**14** Daisy, a 10-year-old girl, has recently been diagnosed with epilepsy and her neurology specialist would like to start her on gabapentin as an adjunct to her sodium valproate, with an aim to monitor and adjust therapy as necessary. The junior doctor is unsure how to initiate this new agent and asks for your advice.
After determining her body weight as 35 kg, which of the following would be the most appropriate initiation regimen?
For this question you may find it useful to use the monograph for gabapentin in the current version of the BNFC.

- ☐ **A** 300 mg OD on day 1, 300 mg BD on day 2, then 300 mg TDS thereafter
- ☐ **B** 350 mg OD on day 1, 350 mg BD on day 2, then 350 mg TDS thereafter
- ☐ **C** 300 mg TDS on day 1, titrated to response in steps of 300 mg every 2–3 days
- ☐ **D** 350 mg TDS on day 1, titrated to response in steps of 300 mg every 2–3 days
- ☐ **E** None of the above; gabapentin is not suitable for this patient

**15** You are conducting an MUR for one of your patients, Mrs F. Upon asking her how she feels today she says she has been feeling a little under the weather recently after developing a sore throat, which she dismisses as having picked up at work.
Which ONE of her regular medicines, if any, may be causing her sore throat?

- ☐ **A** citalopram 20 mg OM
- ☐ **B** mirtazapine 15 mg ON
- ☐ **C** *Oramorph* 2.5 mL QDS PRN
- ☐ **D** paracetamol 1 g QDS
- ☐ **E** None of the above; she probably caught it at work

**16** You are working as the on-call pharmacist for your hospital and you get a call from one of the nurses, Jenny, on the hyper-acute stroke unit. One of their newly admitted patients, Mr Z, is unable to swallow properly and they would like to know which medicines they can crush to help him take his medicines.
Assuming Mr Z can swallow liquids and purees, which medicine(s) should NOT be crushed or dispersed by Jenny?

- ☐ **A** *Calcichew D3 Forte* tablets
- ☐ **B** digoxin 62.5 mg tablets
- ☐ **C** finasteride 5 mg tablets
- ☐ **D** isosorbide mononitrate 10 mg tablets
- ☐ **E** warfarin 1 mg tablets
- ☐ **F** None of Mr Z's tablets should be crushed

Question 17 concerns Mr T who arrives at your community pharmacy complaining of itchy legs. You invite him into your consultation room to look at his legs and observe the following:

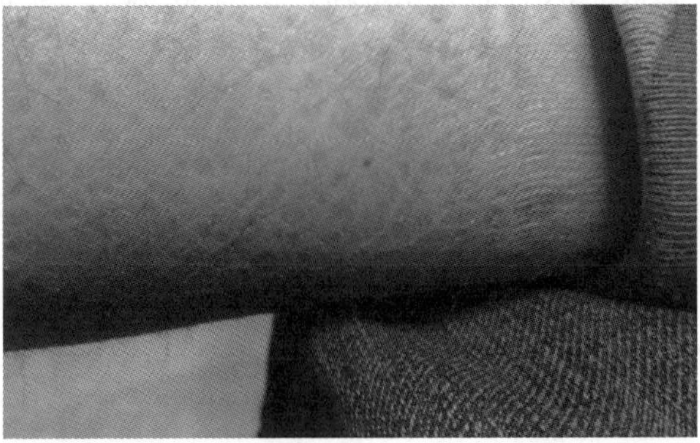

Source: © Skock3/Wikimedia Commons/CC-BY-SA-3

**17** After examining Mr T, what would be the most appropriate course of action?

- ☐ **A** Supply an 'aftersun' cream
- ☐ **B** Supply *Daktacort* cream
- ☐ **C** Supply *Diprobase* cream
- ☐ **D** Refer this patient to his GP
- ☐ **E** Advise patient this is a self-limiting condition

18 You are called by one of the on-call doctors for the haematology wards who has a patient, Mrs W, with an INR of 8.3. They have withheld her warfarin this evening and plan to see how the INR responds tomorrow. However, the nurses have just reported that Mrs W's gums have bled after brushing her teeth, which doesn't normally happen. Which of the following would be the most appropriate action to take?

- ☐ A Give Mrs W a dose of digoxin-specific antibody fragments
- ☐ B Give Mrs W a dose of enoxaparin
- ☐ C Give Mrs W a dose of phytomenadione
- ☐ D Refer Mrs W for dialysis
- ☐ E The warfarin has already been stopped and nothing else needs to be done

19 Mr A comes into your pharmacy to pick up a prescription for lorazepam 0.5 mg QDS. He is well known to you and has been using the lorazepam for anxiety for a number of months. He was listening to the news about the drug driving laws and worries he might get arrested.
If Mr A were to be pulled over, which of the following instances would not be classed as an offence?

- ☐ A His driving is not impaired, he takes his tablets as prescribed and his serum lorazepam concentration is above the limit
- ☐ B His driving is not impaired, he takes his tablets as he feels best suits him and his serum lorazepam concentration is above the limit
- ☐ C His driving is impaired, he takes his tablets as prescribed and his serum lorazepam concentration is above the limit
- ☐ D His driving is impaired, he takes his tablets as he feels best suits him and his serum lorazepam concentration is above the limit
- ☐ E All of the above result in a criminal offence because his lorazepam serum concentrations are above the allowed limit

20 Mrs L is one of the patients on your oncology ward and has recently had her analgesia increased to *OxyContin* (oxycodone MR) 20 mg BD alongside *Oxynorm* (oxycodone) 5 mg PRN. A few days later, upon inspecting her stool chart, you notice she has not opened her bowels for the past 2 days. You discuss this with the medical team and agree she needs a laxative.
Which of the following options would be most appropriate?

- ☐ A lactulose 10 mL BD PRN
- ☐ B senna 15 mg ON PRN
- ☐ C lactulose 10 mL BD and senna 7.5–15 mg ON PRN
- ☐ D lactulose 10 mL BD and *Movicol* (macrogol powder) 1 sachet ON PRN
- ☐ E Mrs L should be referred for urgent bowel evacuation

21 Miss J is one of your regular patients and this afternoon she comes into your pharmacy to buy some multivitamin tablets. Earlier that morning her GP diagnosed her with a number of vitamin deficiencies, notably A, D, E, and K, but she wasn't prepared to pay another prescription fee as she is on a number of medicines already.
Which of the following of her regular medicines may be causing this vitamin deficiency?

- ☐ A atorvastatin
- ☐ B captopril
- ☐ C metformin
- ☐ D orlistat
- ☐ E None of the above is the likely cause

Questions 22 and 23 concern Mr U, a 45-year-old black man with diabetes who has recently been admitted to your general medical ward after complaining of general ill health over the past few weeks.

22 During your visit to the general medical ward you note that Mr U was started on bisoprolol 10 mg for hypertension by the night team. Why should you be cautious of using bisoprolol to treat Mr U's hypertension?

- ☐ A Mr U has a higher risk of bradycardia
- ☐ B Mr U has a higher risk of syncope
- ☐ C Mr U is unlikely to respond to bisoprolol
- ☐ D Mr U will be at increased risk from hypoglycaemia
- ☐ E Mr U will be at increased risk of respiratory distress

23 While discussing this choice of treatment with the day team, the consultant agrees bisoprolol was a poor choice for this patient.
What should be the first-choice agent to treat Mr U's hypertension?

- ☐ A amlodipine 5 mg OD
- ☐ B bendroflumethiazide 2.5 mg OD
- ☐ C indapamide 1.5 mg OD
- ☐ D losartan 50 mg OD
- ☐ E ramipril 2.5 mg OD

24 Mrs E comes into your community pharmacy to collect her regular prescription. While handing out her medicines you note that she is wearing new tinted spectacles. Upon further questioning you learn she has recently been getting dazzled by car headlights and decided to get her spectacles tinted.
Which of her regular medicines, if any, may have contributed to this?

- ☐ A amiodarone 200 mg OD
- ☐ B aspirin 75 mg OD
- ☐ C atorvastatin 40 mg ON
- ☐ D ramipril 2.5 mg ON
- ☐ E None of the above

25 Mr B is a man on your elderly care ward who is being treated for a fractured bone. While reviewing Mr B's current treatment you note the nurses have reported that whilst his stools are normal in consistency they have darkened and are now a black colour.
Which of Mr B's medicines, if any, is likely to have caused this?

- ☐ A aspirin 75 mg OM
- ☐ B ferrous sulfate 200 mg TDS
- ☐ C itraconazole 200 mg BD
- ☐ D simvastatin 40 mg ON
- ☐ E None of the above; he has probably had a gastrointestinal bleed

Questions 26 and 27 concern Mrs K, a patient on your infectious diseases unit. She has been newly prescribed ciprofloxacin 400 mg BD, which will be continued on discharge via the hospital's OPAT (Outpatient Parenteral Antibiotic Therapy) service.
You may find it useful to consult the SPC for IV ciprofloxacin to answer these questions: http://www.medicines.org.uk/emc/medicine/2536.

**26** Mrs K is on a number of antimicrobial therapies over the course of each day and the nursing staff wish to reduce the burden this has on Mrs K and the OPAT team.
When asked what the quickest infusion time for ciprofloxacin is, what would you advise?

- ☐ **A** IV infusion over 10 minutes
- ☐ **B** IV infusion over 30 minutes
- ☐ **C** IV infusion over 60 minutes
- ☐ **D** IV infusion over 120 minutes
- ☐ **E** Continuous IV infusion over 24 hours

**27** The OPAT team would also like to lock Mrs K's IV cannula with *Hepsal* (heparinised saline 50 units/mL) to maintain its patency.
Which of the following would be the least appropriate to advise the OPAT team to do?

- ☐ **A** Flush and lock the line with 10 ml *Hepsal*
- ☐ **B** Flush line with 10 mL 5% glucose then lock the line with 10 mL *Hepsal*
- ☐ **C** Flush line with 10 mL 0.9% sodium chloride then lock the line with 10 mL *Hepsal*
- ☐ **D** Flush line with 10 mL water for injections then lock the line with 10 mL *Hepsal*
- ☐ **E** None of the above is suitable advice

**28** You are compiling a drug history for a new patient, Mr Y, who has been admitted onto your acute medical admissions unit. While going through the medicines he has brought in with him you note two of them, *Tazko* and *Furesis*, were obtained in Finland while visiting family. You are unsure what these medicines are and need to find out.
Which of the following resources would you consult first?

- ☐ **A** *AHFS Drug Information*
- ☐ **B** *British National Formulary*
- ☐ **C** *Martindale: The Complete Drug Reference*
- ☐ **D** *Medicines Ethics and Practice Guide*
- ☐ **E** *Remington: The Science and Practice of Pharmacy*

29 Josh is a 14-year-old boy on your gastrointestinal surgery ward who has just come round from anaesthetic after having a partial ileal resection. Josh's father approaches you and the paediatric SHO mentioning that Josh is feeling sick and wondered if there was something he could have. Which of the following should NOT be prescribed for Josh?

- ☐ A cyclizine
- ☐ B domperidone
- ☐ C metoclopramide
- ☐ D ondansetron
- ☐ E promethazine

30 Mrs Q comes into your community pharmacy with her 2-month-old son Patrice because she wants to talk to you about Patrice's flaky scalp. Upon questioning you determine that her son hasn't been itching, the flakes are not elsewhere on his body, and he is feeding well. You ask to look at this scalp and observe the following:

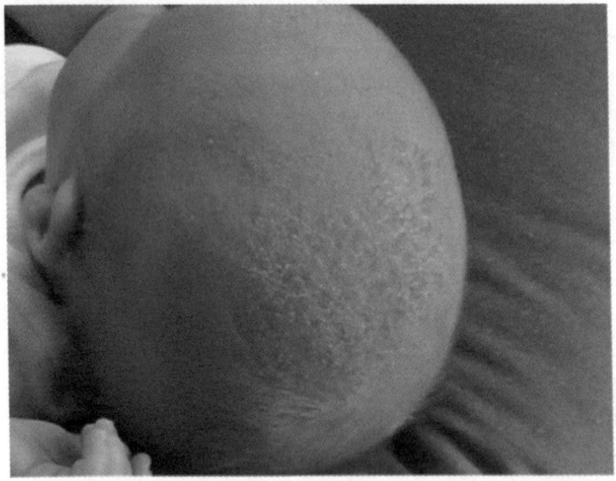

Source: © Starfoxy~commonswiki/Wikimedia Commons/CC-BY-SA-3.0

Which of the following would be the most appropriate course of action to take?

- ☐ A Advise Mrs Q to massage olive oil onto Patrice's scalp
- ☐ B Advise Mrs Q to apply clotrimazole 1% cream to Patrice's scalp
- ☐ C Advise Mrs Q to apply hydrocortisone 0.5% cream to Patrice's scalp
- ☐ D Advise Mrs Q to take Patrice to see their GP
- ☐ E Advise Mrs Q to take Patrice to A&E

## SECTION B

Babir Malik

1 You are counselling Mrs P, a 65-year-old woman, who has just been diagnosed with postmenopausal osteoporosis. She has been prescribed:

Alendronic acid 70 mg (4)
Take ONE tablet ONCE weekly on the same day

Which ONE of the following is the most appropriate piece of advice to give to Mrs P?

- ☐ A Chew tablets
- ☐ B Stand or sit upright for at least 30 minutes after administration
- ☐ C Take at least 15 minutes before another oral medication
- ☐ D Take at night
- ☐ E Take with milk

2 Flurbiprofen (*Strefen*) is available OTC for the symptomatic relief of sore throats for adults, the elderly and children over the age of 12 years. Which ONE of the following drugs would be most appropriate for use alongside flurbiprofen?

- ☐ A aspirin 75 mg
- ☐ B dabigatran
- ☐ C lithium
- ☐ D methotrexate
- ☐ E pizotifen

3 Many of the principles behind the seven principles of the code of ethics come from the work done by Beauchamp and Childress from Georgetown, USA (Beauchamp TL, Childress JF. *Principles of Biomedical Ethics*, 6th edn. New York: Oxford University Press, 2008).
Which of the following is ONE of Beauchamp and Childress's principles of biomedical ethics?

- ☐ A equity
- ☐ B integrity
- ☐ C freedom
- ☐ D justice
- ☐ E liberty

4 Mrs P is 80 years old, lives by herself and can't read. She has carers who come in to her house twice a day. She is prescribed warfarin and wants to know what the correct colours for each of her warfarin tablets are.

- ☐ A 1 mg brown, 3 mg pink and 5 mg blue
- ☐ B 1 mg pink, 3 mg blue and 5 mg brown
- ☐ C 1 mg blue, 3 mg brown and 5 mg pink
- ☐ D 1 mg brown, 3 mg blue and 5 mg pink
- ☐ E 1 mg blue, 3 mg pink and 5 mg brown

5 Miss W, an 18-year-old young woman, lives next door to your pharmacy and comes in screaming and seeking advice for a burn on her left arm. She received the burn 2 minutes ago from her hair straighteners. The burn is smaller than a 1-inch square and is not a full-thickness burn. It has just started blistering.
Which ONE of the following is the most appropriate thing to do first?

- ☐ A Apply a burn cream such as *Acriflex*
- ☐ B Burst the blister
- ☐ C Cool the burn
- ☐ D Dress the burn
- ☐ E Ring for an ambulance

6 Mrs L, a 45-year-old woman, brings in a prescription for a urinary tract infection:

Trimethoprim 200 mg (6)
Take ONE tablet TWICE daily

You recall that she is also taking another medicine that interacts and you decide to discuss this with her GP.
Which ONE of the following should NOT be used with trimethoprim?

- ☐ A digoxin
- ☐ B enalapril
- ☐ C lithium
- ☐ D methotrexate
- ☐ E warfarin

7 A local GP is told by a patient about a new drug licensed for premature ejaculation. He rings you to ask what it is called.

- ☐ A dapoxetine
- ☐ B duloxetine
- ☐ C fluoxetine
- ☐ D paroxetine
- ☐ E reboxetine

Questions 8–10 relate to ear preparations.

8 Sandra, a practice nurse, rings you up to ask you about otitis externa. Which ONE of these corticosteroids is NOT used to treat inflammation and eczema in otitis externa?

☐ A alclometasone
☐ B betamethasone sodium phosphate
☐ C dexamethasone
☐ D flumetasone pivalate
☐ E prednisolone sodium phosphate

9 Mrs CS presents with a stain on her cheek and white shirt. She says it was caused by her ear drops.
Which ONE of the following ear drop preparations is it likely to be?

☐ A chloramphenicol
☐ B clioquinol
☐ C clotrimazole
☐ D framycetin sulfate
☐ E gentamicin

10 Mrs AJ is a 35-year-old Polish woman. She has a nut allergy.
Which ONE of these ear drops for wax should NOT be recommended for Mrs AJ?

☐ A chlorobutanol 5%, arachis oil 57.3% (*Cerumol*)
☐ B urea–hydrogen peroxide complex 5% in glycerol (*Exterol*)
☐ C olive oil
☐ D urea–hydrogen peroxide 5% (*Otex*)
☐ E sodium bicarbonate

11 Peter wants to buy an emollient that doesn't contain urea for his fiancée, Katie, as she read in a magazine that it's not good for the skin.
Which ONE would be the most appropriate?

☐ A *Aquadrate*
☐ B *Balneum*
☐ C *Calmurid*
☐ D *E45 Itch Relief* cream
☐ E *Hydromol*

12 Dr K is concerned about the unavailability of clobetasone butyrate 0.05% (*Eumovate*) and wants you to recommend an alternative steroid cream with a similar potency.
Which ONE is the most suitable?

☐ A alcometasone dipropionate 0.05% (*Modrasone*)
☐ B betamethasone dipropionate 0.05% (*Diprosone*)
☐ C betamethasone valerate 0.1% (*Betnovate*)
☐ D fluticasone propionate 0.05% (*Cutivate*)
☐ E mometasone furoate 0.1% (*Elocon*)

13 Miss C was taking oxybutynin for urinary incontinence but got some of the antimuscarinic side-effects. She wants you to recommend a drug that won't cause those side-effects which she can ask her GP to prescribe.
Which ONE would be the most suitable?

☐ A darifenacin
☐ B fesoterodine
☐ C mirabegron
☐ D propiverine
☐ E solfenacin

14 Mr M has oral thrush and wants to buy some *Daktarin* oral gel. He gives you his repeat slip.
Which ONE of his medications is contraindicated with miconazole?

☐ A bisoprolol
☐ B calcium carbonate 1.25 g/cholecalciferol 10 mcg
☐ C diclofenac
☐ D ezetimibe
☐ E simvastatin

15 Mr S, a 26-year-old builder, presents with a mild flare-up of his eczema on his arms.
Which ONE of the following could be sold to him OTC?

☐ A 0.1% hydrocortisone and 0.05% clobetasone butyrate
☐ B 0.1% hydrocortisone and 0.05% clobetasol propionate
☐ C 0.5% hydrocortisone and 0.05% clobetasone butyrate
☐ D 1% hydrocortisone and 0.05% clobetasol propionate
☐ E 1% hydrocortisone and 0.05% clobetasone butyrate

Questions 16 and 17 relate to haemorrhoid preparations.

**16** Miss S, a 26-year-old woman, would like to buy a preparation for haemorrhoids that contains hydrocortisone.
Which ONE of the following statements about hydrocortisone acetate is false?

- ☐ A Haemorrhoidal preparations containing hydrocortisone are available as P medicines
- ☐ B They should be used only in patients over 10 years of age
- ☐ C They should not be used during pregnancy or breastfeeding
- ☐ D They should not be used for more than 7 days
- ☐ E They should not be recommended to new sufferers who have not consulted their doctor

**17** Miss S also asks what each ingredient does in different haemorrhoid preparations.
Which ONE of the following ingredients in haemorrhoid preparations is classed as an astringent?

- ☐ A bismuth oxide
- ☐ B cinchocaine
- ☐ C mucopolysaccharide polysulfate
- ☐ D shark liver oil
- ☐ E yeast cell extract

**18** Mrs PS is 45 years old and would like to buy an antacid. She is not pregnant. She has had her symptoms before.
Which ONE of the following list of disadvantages of antacids is false?

- ☐ A Bismuth salicylate can cause blackening of the faeces
- ☐ B Calcium carbonate can cause constipation
- ☐ C Magnesium hydroxide can cause diarrhoea
- ☐ D Potassium bicarbonate can cause hypokalaemia
- ☐ E Sodium bicarbonate is absorbed systemically

**19** Mr SD asks to speak to you in private. He has scabies and would like a suitable preparation. You show him a tube of permethrin 5% (*Lyclear*) cream and counsel him.
How long should Mr D leave the cream on for?

- ☐ A 1–2 hours
- ☐ B 3–4 hours
- ☐ C 6–8 hours
- ☐ D 8–12 hours
- ☐ E 24 hours

20 Miss SZ would like something for athlete's foot. She is not diabetic and wants an easy fix as she works long hours.
Which ONE of the following is available as a one-dose preparation?

- ☐ A imidazole
- ☐ B griseofulvin
- ☐ C terbinafine
- ☐ D tolnaftate
- ☐ E undecenoates

21 Miss PB has been prescribed colestipol by her nurse prescriber. She wants to know when she should take her other medicines in relation to colestipol.

- ☐ A 1 hour before or 1 hour after
- ☐ B 1 hour before or 4 hours after
- ☐ C 2 hours before or 4 hours after
- ☐ D 30 minutes before or 1 hour after
- ☐ E 30 minutes before or 4 hours after

22 Suzanne, your counter assistant, is undertaking her OTC course. She wants to know what the difference is between *Dioralyte* and *Dioralyte Relief*?

- ☐ A flavour
- ☐ B price
- ☐ C strength
- ☐ D *Dioralyte Relief* contains rice
- ☐ E *Dioralyte Relief* contains flour

23 Mr HM brings in his 6-month-old infant who has had diarrhoea for 5 days.
Which ONE is the most appropriate course of action?

- ☐ A Recommend loperamide
- ☐ B Recommend *Dioralyte*
- ☐ C Recommend *Dioralyte* and refer to GP
- ☐ D Refer to GP for a routine appointment
- ☐ E Send to A&E

**24** Vladimir brings a prescription from Poland to your pharmacy. Which ONE of these schedules of controlled drugs can be dispensed in the UK when prescribed by a doctor, dentist, prescribing pharmacist or prescribing nurse registered in an EE country or Switzerland?

- ☐ **A** Medicinal products without a marketing authorisation in the UK
- ☐ **B** Schedule 1
- ☐ **C** Schedule 2
- ☐ **D** Schedule 3
- ☐ **E** Schedule 4

**25** Mrs OP presents in the pharmacy and wants something for IBS. Which ONE of the following symptoms would lead to a referral to the GP?

- ☐ **A** abdominal pain
- ☐ **B** bloating
- ☐ **C** constipation
- ☐ **D** diarrhoea
- ☐ **E** vomiting

**26** Mr NS, a 25-year-old man, has suffered with dandruff since he was a teenager but has never spoke to a healthcare professional about it. Which ONE of these treatments is NOT indicated for dandruff and seborrhoeic dermatitis?

- ☐ **A** acetic acid
- ☐ **B** coal tar
- ☐ **C** ketoconazole
- ☐ **D** pyrithione zinc
- ☐ **E** selenium sulfide

**27** Which ONE of these OTC drugs with its accompanying minimum age for OTC use is NOT correct?

- ☐ **A** amorolfine: 18 years
- ☐ **B** chloramphenicol: 2 years
- ☐ **C** hydrocortisone cream: 10 years
- ☐ **D** levonorgestrel: 16 years
- ☐ **E** naproxen: 16 years

28 Miss SD presents a prescription for isotretinoin. The prescription indicates that a pregnancy test was negative.
Under the pregnancy prevention programme, prescriptions for isotretinoin are valid for how many days?

☐ A 1
☐ B 7
☐ C 28
☐ D 30
☐ E 60

Questions 29–31 relate to motion sickness medication. Mr B asks your advice about the advantages and disadvantages of the available options.

29 Which ONE of the following has a 24-hour duration of action?

☐ A cinnarizine (*Stugeron* 15)
☐ B hyoscine (*Joy Rides*)
☐ C hyoscine (*Kwells*)
☐ D promethazine hydrochloride (*Phenergan*)
☐ E promethazine teoclate (*Avomine*)

30 Which ONE causes the most sedation?

☐ A cinnarizine (*Stugeron* 15)
☐ B hyoscine (*Joy Rides*)
☐ C hyoscine (*Kwells*)
☐ D promethazine hydrochloride (*Phenergan*)
☐ E promethazine teoclate (*Avomine*)

31 Which ONE would be most suitable for a 6-hour journey?

☐ A cinnarizine (*Stugeron* 15)
☐ B hyoscine (*Joy Rides*)
☐ C hyoscine (*Kwells*)
☐ D promethazine hydrochloride (*Phenergan*)
☐ E promethazine teoclate (*Avomine*)

Questions 32–34 relate to *Regaine for Men Extra Strength* 5%. Mr K is 45 years old and would like some advice on the product.
You may find it useful to consult the SPC for this product to answer these questions: https://www.medicines.org.uk/emc/medicine/16535.

**32** He wants to know for how long the effects last in his body.
Following cessation of dosing, approximately 95% of topically applied minoxidil will be eliminated within how many days?

- ☐ **A** 1
- ☐ **B** 2
- ☐ **C** 3
- ☐ **D** 4
- ☐ **E** 5

**33** He asks how much he can use in a day.
What's the maximum daily dosage?

- ☐ **A** 2 mL
- ☐ **B** 5 mL
- ☐ **C** 20 mL
- ☐ **D** 50 mL
- ☐ **E** 100 mL

**34** The answer to question 33 is equivalent to the maximum recommended adult dose for oral minoxidil administration in the treatment of hypertension.
How much is this in milligrams?

- ☐ **A** 1 mg
- ☐ **B** 10 mg
- ☐ **C** 100 mg
- ☐ **D** 1000 mg
- ☐ **E** 10 000 mg

Questions 35–37 relate to *Nytol One-A-Night*. Mrs M, a 55-year-old woman, is asking for advice.
You may find it useful to consult the SPC for this product to answer these questions: https://www.medicines.org.uk/emc/medicine/19778.

**35** You ask her if she has any medical conditions.
*Nytol One-A-Night* is NOT cautioned in which of the following?

- ☐ **A** asthma
- ☐ **B** bronchitis
- ☐ **C** COPD
- ☐ **D** epilepsy
- ☐ **E** open-angle glaucoma

**36** What percentage of a single dose is excreted unchanged in urine?

☐ A 1%
☐ B 2%
☐ C 3%
☐ D 4%
☐ E 5%

**37** She asks you after how many hours of a single dose will the sedative effect be at its maximum.

☐ A 1 hour
☐ B 2 hour
☐ C 1–2 hours
☐ D 1–3 hours
☐ E 1–4 hours

**38** You are discussing OTC medicines with your pre-registration pharmacist.
Which ONE of the following patients does NOT need to be referred to their doctor?

☐ A 4-month-old infant needing *Daktarin Sugar Free Oral Gel*
☐ B 11-month-old infant needing *Piriton* syrup
☐ C 15-year-old female wanting *Germoloids* HC spray
☐ D 17-year-old male wanting *Beconase Hayfever Relief* nasal spray
☐ E 66-year-old male wanting *Regaine for Men Extra Strength*

**39** A pharmaceutical representative comes in to talk to you about *Nexium Control*.
Which ONE of the following statements about *Nexium Control* is true?

☐ A It is the brand for OTC omeprazole
☐ B It is available as a 20 mg tablet
☐ C The dose is 20 mg BD
☐ D It is licensed for stomach ulcers
☐ E It is available only from pharmacies

40 Miss Taylor brings in her 9-month-old child who has tiny vesicles that are filled with fluid. They are surrounded by red areas on the trunk and are all over. The rash developed 3 days ago and appears to be getting worse. The child was restless for a few days before the rash appeared. The child is on no other medication and is healthy.
Which ONE is the most appropriate course of action?

- ☐ A No action is needed
- ☐ B Recommend an appropriate product
- ☐ C Recommend appropriate lifestyle advice
- ☐ D Refer to A&E
- ☐ E Refer to GP

## SECTION C

Oksana Pyzik

1 Miss JT is 61 years old and is going on a cruise with her husband for 2 weeks. She has no allergies but has suffered from severe seasickness in the past.
Which ONE of the following is the most effective treatment for nausea and vomiting associated with motion sickness?

- ☐ A chlorpromazine hydrochloride
- ☐ B hyoscine hydrobromide
- ☐ C ondansetron
- ☐ D prochlorperazine
- ☐ E promethazine

2 Mr L comes into the pharmacy seeking advice for an itchy, inflamed and painful external right ear. He is an avid swimmer and has had similar problems before.
Which ONE of the following is NOT a referral point for his condition?

- ☐ A profuse mucopurulent discharge
- ☐ B symptoms lasting for 4 or more days without improvement
- ☐ C pain on palpitation of the mastoid area
- ☐ D fever lasting 24 hours
- ☐ E conductive hearing loss

Questions 3–5 refer to the legal requirements surrounding the advertisement of medicines in the UK.

3 Which ONE of the following statements regarding the advertisement of medicines is NOT true?

- ☐ A Websites should not have POM names in the address
- ☐ B POMs may not be advertised
- ☐ C Promotional claims of unlicensed medicines may not be included in adverts
- ☐ D The advertising of medicines is regulated by the GPhC
- ☐ E The MHRA has the power to vet medicines advertisements in advance of publication

4 Which ONE of the following is an example of primary literature?

- ☐ A systematic reviews
- ☐ B original clinical trials
- ☐ C special reports
- ☐ D letters to editor
- ☐ E journal periodicals

5 Which ONE of the following is NOT an example of an activity defined as the advertising of medicines?

- ☐ A Visits by medical sales representatives
- ☐ B Supply of samples to healthcare professionals
- ☐ C Provision of inducements to prescribe
- ☐ D Sponsorship of meetings
- ☐ E Supply of health promotional material surrounding disease states

6 Miss O is travelling to Peru to climb Machu Picchu and requires the yellow fever vaccine.
For how long will she have immunity before requiring re-vaccination?

- ☐ A 2 years
- ☐ B 3 years
- ☐ C 5 years
- ☐ D 10 years
- ☐ E 15 years

7 Mr U is a 48-year-old man who presents at your community pharmacy seeking advice about the red patches on his knees and elbows. Upon examination the lesions appear salmon pink with silvery white scales. When the scales on the surface of the plaque are gently removed and the lesion is rubbed, it reveals pinpoint bleeding from the superficial dilated capillaries.
Which form of psoriasis is the most likely cause of Mr U's symptoms?

- ☐ A erythrodermic
- ☐ B guttate
- ☐ C plaque
- ☐ D pustular
- ☐ E seborrhoeic

8 Miss P is suffering from acute infectious diarrhoea caused by *Shigella*. Which ONE of the following is NOT appropriate advice to give?

- ☐ A Avoid food intake for at least 6 hours
- ☐ B Take small frequent sips of water then slowly increase fluid intake
- ☐ C Use glucose solutions such as soda to settle the stomach and decrease the number of stools
- ☐ D It is a self-limiting condition and therefore no treatment is necessary
- ☐ E If symptoms are severe or persistent, doxycycline may be prescribed for a 7-day course

9 Mr S is a 69-year-old man who has been diagnosed with hypertension and arrhythmia. As the hospital pharmacist on the cardiac ward, you have counselled him on his newly prescribed medicines. The pre-registration pharmacist whom you are training has further questions regarding myocardial oxygen demand.
Which ONE of the following is least likely to increase myocardial oxygen demand?

- ☐ A cold temperatures
- ☐ B exercise
- ☐ C isoprenaline
- ☐ D metoprolol
- ☐ E smoking

10 Mrs G presents at the pharmacy with constipation and asks you what she can take to relieve her symptoms as quickly as possible.
Which ONE of the following OTC products has the quickest onset of action in the treatment of acute constipation?

- ☐ A bisacodyl
- ☐ B docusate sodium
- ☐ C ispaghula husk
- ☐ D lactulose
- ☐ E loperamide

**11** Miss ZM has just been diagnosed with recurrent migraine headaches and has been prescribed sumatriptan 100 mg for treatment of attacks. Which ONE of the following pre-existing conditions is contraindicated for the use of sumatriptan in this patient?

- ☐ A gouty arthritis
- ☐ B irritable bowel syndrome
- ☐ C ischaemic heart disease
- ☐ D mild liver impairment
- ☐ E renal failure

**12** Mrs T's 12-year-old son has permanent yellow-to-greyish stains on his teeth. She tells you that the doctor explained that a medicine was responsible for the pigmentation.
Which ONE of the following medicines is most likely to have caused *intrinsic staining* of the teeth?

- ☐ A chlorhexidine mouthwash
- ☐ B co-amoxiclav suspension
- ☐ C fluoride drops
- ☐ D sodium feredetate elixir
- ☐ E tetracycline tablets

**13** Miss U is a 33-year-old woman who suffers from recurrent aphthous ulcers that she describes as very painful. You check her patient medication record and notice that she has been taking the prescribed and OTC medicines below although not concomitantly.
Which ONE of the following medicines is least likely to cause ulceration of the oral mucosa?

- ☐ A aspirin
- ☐ B ibuprofen
- ☐ C methotrexate
- ☐ D propranolol
- ☐ E ramipril

**14** Mrs V is 55 years old and has been diagnosed with severe heart failure. She has been prescribed spironolactone as an adjunct treatment to her existing therapy.
Which ONE of the following describes the mechanism of action of spironolactone in heart failure?

- ☐ A positive inotropic effect
- ☐ B positive chronotropic effect
- ☐ C negative inotropic effect
- ☐ D aldosterone antagonism
- ☐ E angiotensin II blockade

**15** The pharmacy you are working at is looking to expand its pharmacy provision services to compete with other local pharmacies.
Under the NHS Pharmacy contract, which ONE of the following is an example of an advanced service?

- ☐ A minor ailment service
- ☐ B needle and syringe exchange
- ☐ C medicines use review
- ☐ D public health
- ☐ E patient group directions

**16** Mr E has been rushed to accident and emergency at your local hospital due to an overdose of paracetamol tablets.
Which of the following symptoms is most characteristic of paracetamol toxicity?

- ☐ A profound vasoconstriction and hyperventilation
- ☐ B central nervous system stimulation and seizures
- ☐ C diarrhoea and severe abdominal cramping
- ☐ D severe hepatocellular necrosis
- ☐ E renal tubular necrosis

**17** Mr D has been prescribed warfarin and has also been seeking complementary and alternative therapies, such as treatment with vitamins, to improve his health.
Which ONE of the following vitamins should Mr D avoid?

- ☐ A vitamin A
- ☐ B vitamin B
- ☐ C vitamin D
- ☐ D vitamin E
- ☐ E vitamin K

18 Mr V is admitted to hospital with the following symptoms: hypotension, arrhythmias and complete heart block. Parenteral calcium is used as an antidote.
Mr V is being treated for which of the following medical emergencies?

- ☐ A aspirin overdose
- ☐ B verapamil overdose
- ☐ C hypokalaemia
- ☐ D cocaine intoxication
- ☐ E heroin overdose

19 Mrs F is a 41-year-old woman undergoing treatment for lymphomatous meningitis.
Which ONE of the following chemotherapy agents can be administered intrathecally?

- ☐ A cytarabine
- ☐ B vinblastine
- ☐ C vincristine
- ☐ D vindesine
- ☐ E vinflunine

20 Mrs C has come to your pharmacy seeking advice for her 2-year-old son who is suffering from a cough and cold.
Which ONE of the following classes of ingredients is safe to recommend to Mrs C for her son?

- ☐ A antitussives
- ☐ B antihistamines
- ☐ C demulcents
- ☐ D nasal decongestants
- ☐ E expectorants

21 Prochaska and DiClemente's cycle of change is often used in community pharmacy as a model to help pharmacists engage with patients who wish to stop smoking.
Which ONE of the following stages is NOT part of the cycle of change?

- ☐ A action
- ☐ B contemplation
- ☐ C evaluation
- ☐ D precontemplation
- ☐ E preparation

22 A mother enquires about what product she can purchase for her 6-year-old son. He has several insect bites after a school camping trip. He complains that the bites are itchy and inflamed, and continuously scratches the area, leading to bleeding.
Which ONE of the following products may NOT be supplied for the treatment of insect bites and stings in this case?

- ☐ A ammonia 3.5% w/w (*AfterBite*)
- ☐ B chlorphenamine (*Piriton*)
- ☐ C crotamiton (*Eurax*)
- ☐ D hydrocortisone (*Dermacort*)
- ☐ E lidocaine (*Dermidex*)

23 Which ONE of the following symptoms is NOT a sign of chlamydia infection?

- ☐ A vulvovaginal sores
- ☐ B pain in the lower abdomen
- ☐ C vaginal bleeding during sexual intercourse
- ☐ D dysuria
- ☐ E penile discharge

24 In which of the following cases may tamsulosin (*Flomax*) be supplied OTC?

- ☐ A Symptoms that have been present for 2 weeks
- ☐ B Patients with postural hypotension
- ☐ C Patients with unstable diabetes
- ☐ D Patients undergoing cataract surgery
- ☐ E Patients with enlarged prostate gland

25 Miss H presents at your local pharmacy and would like to purchase tranexamic acid for her heavy periods.
Which ONE of the following statements regarding treatment with tranexamic acid is NOT true?

- ☐ A Treatment with tranexamic acid is initiated only once heavy bleeding has started
- ☐ B The recommended dosage is two tablets three times daily for a maximum of 4 days
- ☐ C May be used for women with heavy periods from the age of 16
- ☐ D May not be used by women taking the oral contraceptive pill
- ☐ E May not be used by women having more than 3 days of individual variability in their menstrual cycle periods

26 Mr E has just purchased contact lenses. He is looking for a contact lens solution that may be used to clean and moisten the surface of the contact lens while the lens is still in the eye.
Which ONE of the following contact lens solutions is most appropriate for application in the eye?

- ☐ A rewetting solution
- ☐ B wetting solution
- ☐ C cleaning solution
- ☐ D soaking solution
- ☐ E conditioning solution

27 Mrs T is a 59-year-old woman who has been prescribed amiodarone. She has been advised by the hospital pharmacist that this medicine may cause phototoxicity. In addition to keeping out of the sun, she asks for a sunscreen just in case as the summer months are approaching.
Which ONE of the following sunscreen agents and active ingredients will NOT prevent a drug-induced photosensitivity reaction?

- ☐ A octyl methoxycinnamate and homosalate
- ☐ B padimate O and avobenzone
- ☐ C padimate O and oxybenzone
- ☐ D titanium dioxide
- ☐ E zinc oxide

28 Mr M is a 43-year-old man of Pakistani origin who has been prescribed sitagliptin (*Januvia*) as an adjunct for better control of his condition.
Which ONE of the following statements regarding sitagliptin (*Januvia*) is NOT correct?

- ☐ A It is an inhibitor of dipeptidyl peptidase enzyme (DPP-4) which enhances the incretin hormone
- ☐ B It can cause hypoglycaemia with sulfonylureas
- ☐ C It is not appropriate for use in type 1 diabetes
- ☐ D It can be taken with or without food
- ☐ E It should be continued only if HbA1c concentration is reduced by at least 5 percentage points within 6 months of starting treatment

29 Mr A has developed shin splints from high-interval training, including sprints.
Which of the following would you NOT recommend within the first 48 hours following a sports injury?

- ☐ A compression
- ☐ B elevation
- ☐ C heat
- ☐ D ice
- ☐ E rest

30 Mr Q is rushed to A&E at your local hospital for emergency treatment of poisoning. He presents with hyperventilation, vomiting, tinnitus, deafness, sweating and metabolic acidosis.
Which ONE of the following medicines has Mr Q overdosed on based on his presenting symptoms?

- ☐ A aspirin
- ☐ B ethylene glycol
- ☐ C lead
- ☐ D methadone
- ☐ E paracetamol

31 Which ONE of the following actions is least likely to reduce the incidence of a dispensing error occurring?

- ☐ A Checking patient's name, address and date of birth
- ☐ B Checking name of the prescribed medicine
- ☐ C Checking prescribed strength of medicine
- ☐ D Checking directions for use
- ☐ E Checking manufacturer's name

32 A 53-year-old woman with breast cancer has had a total mastectomy. She has been prescribed tamoxifen for positive oestrogen receptors on the tumour. Her medical records indicate that she has also been taking warfarin.
Which ONE of the following counselling points will you communicate to the patient?

- ☐ A Tamoxifen reduces the risk of endometrial cancer
- ☐ B Tamoxifen interacts with warfarin as it reduces its efficacy
- ☐ C Take at night to reduce symptoms of hot flushes
- ☐ D Take on alternate days
- ☐ E Report to hospital immediately if there is any redness, pain or swelling of the leg

33 Miss A comes to collect her prescription for benzoyl peroxide gel and asks what other measures she can take to reduce her facial acne. Which ONE of the following counselling points will you NOT include in your consultation as the pharmacist?

- ☐ A Do not squeeze acne lesions
- ☐ B Exposure to sunlight minimises acne lesions
- ☐ C Apply gel once or twice daily to the whole face, not just to the active lesions
- ☐ D Use water-based non-comedogenic cosmetics
- ☐ E Benzoyl peroxide has a potent bleaching effect

34 Miss J is 30 years old and in the first trimester of her pregnancy. She presents to the pharmacy with sneezing, rhinorrhoea and nasal itching, which started 3 days ago. She feels miserable and symptoms worsen when she cleans the house. She is also taking calcium carbonate and docusate sodium.
Which ONE of the following would be the best recommendation for the treatment of Miss J's symptoms?

- ☐ A *Breathe Right* nasal strips
- ☐ B chlorphenamine
- ☐ C hydroxyzine
- ☐ D intranasal sodium cromoglicate
- ☐ E pseudoephedrine

35 Mr N is a 49-year-old lorry driver. He has been prescribed a new medicine and is concerned that it might prevent him from working. Which ONE of the following medicines may affect driving and performance of skilled tasks?

- ☐ A danazol
- ☐ B mifepristone
- ☐ C misoprostol
- ☐ D tadalafil
- ☐ E tamsulosin

36 Which ONE of the following medicines is NOT available on an NHS prescription?

- ☐ A danazol
- ☐ B dimeticone
- ☐ C malathion
- ☐ D minoxidil 5%
- ☐ E permethrin

37 Mrs A presents at your pharmacy with a 6-month-old child who is crying in a high-pitch tone. You notice that the child is clenching her fists and drawing up her legs. Mrs A explains that her child has been crying excessively frequently and she is looking for a treatment to help soothe the baby.
Which ONE of the following medicines would it be most appropriate to recommend?

☐ A aspirin
☐ B ibuprofen suspension
☐ C magnesium trisilicate
☐ D paracetamol suspension
☐ E simeticone

38 Mr S is a 71-year-old man who was recently been prescribed a new medicine. He is deeply concerned as his urine is now brown in colour.
Which ONE of the following medicines is most likely to have caused his urine to become brown in colour?

☐ A amitriptyline
☐ B metronidazole
☐ C nitrofurantoin
☐ D rifampicin
☐ E zafirlukast

39 Mrs R has been prescribed clindamycin for the treatment of osteomyelitis. She comes into the pharmacy as she has developed diarrhoea and has been to the toilet four times this morning.
Which ONE of the following is the most appropriate course of action for Mrs R?

☐ A Advise her to purchase loperamide capsules
☐ B Advise her to purchase oral rehydration salts
☐ C Advise her to purchase kaolin and morphine mixture
☐ D Advise her that the condition is self-limiting and should resolve on its own
☐ E Advise her to discontinue treatment and contact GP immediately

**40** Mrs A is a 46-year-old woman who has suffered a minor stroke and has been admitted to hospital. Her records indicate a history of migraine with aura and type 2 diabetes.
Which ONE of her following medicines should be discontinued?

- ☐ A enoxaparin
- ☐ B *NovoMix 30*
- ☐ C metformin
- ☐ D trimethoprim
- ☐ E verapamil

Questions 41–43 relate to the following scenario:

Mr W is 58 years old and suffers from high cholesterol, hypertension and type 2 diabetes. At his last review, the GP prescribed *Janumet* 50 mg/1000 mg. You check his notes and see his weight is 88 kg and his height is 1.6 m. His other medications include:

atorvastatin 40 mg OD
tolbutamide 500 mg TDS
*Zimovane* 7.5 mg ON

Questions 41–43 refer to the following SPC: https://www.medicines.org.uk/emc/medicine/23111

**41** Mr W is admitted to hospital for surgery. He is due to undergo an appendectomy. You review his drug chart to make recommendations regarding his current medicines to the consultant.
Which of the following is the most appropriate advice to give regarding *Janumet*?

- ☐ A Monitor plasma glucose levels and do not discontinue
- ☐ B Discontinue treatment 24 hours before surgery
- ☐ C Discontinue treatment 24 hours before surgery and do not resume until 24 hours after surgery
- ☐ D Discontinue treatment 48 hours before surgery
- ☐ E Discontinue treatment 48 hours before surgery and do not resume until 48 hours after surgery

42 Mr W has been admitted to hospital again for a digital subtraction angiography and requires intravascular administration of iodinated contrast agents.
Why should *Janumet* be discontinued before the administration of iodinated contrast agents via the intravascular route?

- ☐ A No changes required
- ☐ B May induce renal failure associated with lactic acidosis
- ☐ C May induce renal failure associated with angiospasm
- ☐ D May induce hepatic failure associated with lactic acidosis
- ☐ E May induce hepatic failure associated with angiospasm

43 Which of the following is NOT contraindicated with *Janumet*?

- ☐ A alcoholism
- ☐ B breastfeeding
- ☐ C dehydration
- ☐ D hepatic impairment
- ☐ E mild renal impairment

Question 44 refers to the following SPC: https://www.medicines.org.uk/emc/medicine/27165

44 Which of the following side-effects are most commonly associated with *Zimovane*?

- ☐ A dizziness
- ☐ B dysgeusia
- ☐ C dyspnoea
- ☐ D fatigue
- ☐ E headache

Questions 45 and 46 refer to the following SPC: https://www.medicines.org.uk/emc/medicine/26366

45 Which of the following natural products may interact to decrease the efficacy of tolbutamide?

- ☐ A devil's claw
- ☐ B feverfew
- ☐ C ginkgo biloba
- ☐ D saw palmetto
- ☐ E St John's wort

46 Which of the following is NOT appropriate advice to include in your consultation with Mr W regarding tolbutamide?

- ☐ **A** A possible side-effect is blurry vision – if this occurs, do not drive or operate machinery
- ☐ **B** Tolbutamide should not be used as a substitute for diet and exercise
- ☐ **C** Consumption of alcohol may lead to hyperglycaemia
- ☐ **D** See GP if persistent fever or sore throat develops
- ☐ **E** If you have difficulty swallowing you may crush the tablets

## SECTION D

Amar Iqbal

Questions 1–3 relate to Master W, a 3-year-old male who presents with his mother to hospital with a rash on his body that started as red sores on his face 2 days ago. His mother also tells you that he is allergic to penicillin.

1 On examination by the doctor it is noted that Master W has a crusty yellow rash around his mouth and chin, which has spread to his trunk. The rash is causing discomfort and pruritus.
Choose the single most likely condition with which Master W has presented.

- ☐ A chickenpox
- ☐ B heat rash
- ☐ C impetigo
- ☐ D measles
- ☐ E ringworm

2 Which ONE of the following is the most suitable treatment of choice for Master W?

- ☐ A aciclovir
- ☐ B calamine cream
- ☐ C clarithromycin
- ☐ D clotrimazole cream
- ☐ E flucloxacillin

3 Which ONE of the following statements is NOT true regarding the condition Master W has presented with?

- ☐ A It can be caused by a staphylococcal infection
- ☐ B It can be caused by a streptococcal infection
- ☐ C Topical disinfectants are useful in treating it
- ☐ D Topical treatment should be used for up to 10 days
- ☐ E Systemic treatment should be for at least 7 days

Question 4 relates to the supply of medication and devices under the NHS contract based on the following extract taken from the Drug Tariff:

**BORDERLINE SUBSTANCES**

GA AMINOB

For use in the dietary management of glutaric aciduria type 1 (GA1). Suitable from three years.

GA GEL

Type 1 glutaric aciduria.

GALACTOMIN 17

Proven lactose intolerance in pre-school children, galactosaemia and galactokinase deficiency.

GALACTOMIN 19 (FRUCTOSE FORMULA)

Glucose plus galactose intolerance.

GENIUS

See: Gluten-Free Products.

GLANDOSANE

Patients suffering from xerostomia (dry mouth) as a result of having or having undergone radiotherapy or sicca syndrome.

GLUCOSE

For use as an energy supplement in sucrose–isomaltase deficiency.

GLUTAFIN GLUTEN-FREE PRODUCTS

See: Gluten-Free Products.

GLUTAFIN GLUTEN-FREE SELECT PRODUCTS

See: Gluten-Free Products.

(*continued*)

**(continued)**

GLUTEN-FREE PRODUCTS (Not necessarily low protein, lactose or sucrose free)
* For Established Gluten Sensitive Enteropathy with coexisting established wheat sensitivity only

Barkat brown rice pizza crust
Barkat gluten-free biscuits
Barkat gluten-free bread mix
Barkat gluten-free brown rice bread
Barkat gluten-free buckwheat pasta (penne, spirals)
Barkat gluten-free cornflakes
Barkat gluten-free crackers
Barkat gluten-free crispbread
Barkat gluten-free digestive biscuits
Barkat gluten-free flour mix
Barkat gluten-free par-baked baguettes
Barkat gluten-free par-baked country sliced loaf
Barkat gluten-free par-baked rolls
Barkat gluten-free par-baked white bread
Barkat gluten-free par-baked white sliced bread
Barkat gluten-free pasta (alphabet, animal shapes, macaroni, shells, spaghetti, spirals, tagliatelle)
Barkat gluten-free porridge flakes
Barkat gluten-free round crackers
Barkat gluten-free wheat-free multigrain bread
Barkat gluten-free white rice bread
Barkat gluten-free wholemeal sliced bread
Barkat white rice pizza crust
BiAlimenta gluten-free pasta (acini di pepe (pasta grains), formati misti (variety pack), penne, sagnette, spirali (spirals), tubetti)
BiAlimenta gluten-free potato pasta gnocchi
BiAlimenta gluten-free potato pasta perle di gnocchi

***(continued)***

Dietary Specials gluten-free cracker bread
Dietary Specials gluten-free pizza bases
Dietary Specials gluten-free white multigrain sliced loaf
Ener-G gluten-free brown rice bread
Ener-G gluten-free cookies (vanilla flavour)
Ener-G gluten-free dinner rolls
* Ener-G gluten-free pizza bases
Ener-G gluten-free rice loaf
Ener-G gluten-free rice pasta (lasagne, macaroni, small shells, spaghetti, vermicelli)



4 Which ONE of the following statements is NOT true based on the above extract?

- ☐ A A list of borderline substances suitable for dispensing appears in part XV of the Drug Tariff
- ☐ B *Barkat* gluten-free biscuits, when prescribed for patients with coeliac disease, must be endorsed with 'ACBS' on the prescription
- ☐ C *Genius* is a brand of gluten-free products that can be found in the Drug Tariff borderline substances section
- ☐ D *Glandosane* spray can be prescribed for patients with a dry mouth following chemotherapy
- ☐ E Gluten-free products can be described as being lactose free and having a low-protein content

Questions 5 and 6 concern a community pharmacy where you are working as the responsible pharmacist as part of your managerial duties.

5 Which ONE of the following statements is correct in relation to your duties?

- ☐ **A** You cannot make changes to the stores standard operating procedures even if you feel this is necessary to ensure a suitable level of service
- ☐ **B** You have overarching responsibility for the safe and effective running of the store even if you are not present in the store
- ☐ **C** If you leave the store you must remain contactable with the pharmacy staff or arrange for another pharmacist to be available
- ☐ **D** As responsible pharmacist you are allowed to be absent from the store for more than 2 hours in the course of the business day
- ☐ **E** If you are absent from the pharmacy, the counter assistant can sell *Canesten* thrush cream to a female customer who requests it

6 Mr W comes into your pharmacy to confirm whether or not he has been issued the right medication as 'it looks different to his normal tablets'. You take a look and note that the wrong product has been supplied. Which ONE of the following single statements is true?

- ☐ **A** You are unable to rectify the error and supply Mr W with the correct medication
- ☐ **B** It is illegal to supply Mr W any further medication without a new prescription
- ☐ **C** The source of the dispensing error does not need to be investigated
- ☐ **D** Medication errors, even if they do not cause harm, should be reported via the NRLS
- ☐ **E** You must review the dispensing and collection standard operating procedure

Questions 7–9 relate to the following extract taken from a recent clinical letter detailing Master T's current medication:

> Abidec multivitamin drops – 1.2 mL OM
> Azithromycin 250 mg M/W/F each week
> Creon 10 000 unit capsules – up to 32 per day
> Dornase alfa 2.5 mg nebules – 2.5 mg OD
> Salbutamol 100 mcg inhaler – 2 puffs BD
> Fluticasone 50 mcg inhaler – 2 puffs BD
> Vitamin A + D tablets – 1 OM
> Vitamin E 100 mg/mL suspension – 50 units OM

You are working as a pharmacist independent prescriber in your local hospital's respiratory clinic. You are in consultation with Master T, a 14-year-old male, who is accompanied by his mother and father.

7 Using the extract above, choose the single most appropriate condition that the prescribed medication is being used to manage.

- ☐ A asthma
- ☐ B bronchiolitis
- ☐ C croup
- ☐ D cystic fibrosis
- ☐ E pneumonia

8 Master T's parents would like advice on how best to manage his *Creon* capsule administration.
Choose the single most appropriate piece of advice that you should provide.

- ☐ A The capsules should be given on an empty stomach for maximal absorption
- ☐ B The capsules can be opened and mixed with cold milk or apple juice
- ☐ C The capsules should be swallowed whole and not chewed due to an enteric coating
- ☐ D The capsules should be given in equal increments throughout the day
- ☐ E The capsules should be given every 4 hours during daytime hours only

9 During the consultation, Master T's mother asks if you could provide her with a prescription for vitamin E 100 mg/mL suspension, which she is running short of. Vitamin E is available as an unlicensed product. Which ONE of the following statements is NOT true regarding this medication?

☐ A Vitamin E is also known as alfa-tocopherol
☐ B Vitamin E is classed as a fat-soluble vitamin
☐ C Vitamin E is needed due to fat malabsorption
☐ D Vitamin E cannot be prescribed by you
☐ E Vitamin E prescribing carries extra liability

Questions 10–12 concern Mrs Y, a 46-year-old woman weighing 50 kg who is suffering from aspergillosis. Mrs Y is on no regular medication at home and is admitted to hospital for treatment with liposomal amphotericin. Her renal and hepatic functions are normal.
Using the SPC via the following link, https://www.medicines.org.uk/emc/medicine/1236, answer the questions that follow:

10 Which ONE of the following is the most suitable diluent for use as a flush before and after liposomal amphotericin is administered?

☐ A glucose 5%
☐ B heparin sodium (50 units/5 mL)
☐ C sodium chloride 0.45%
☐ D sodium chloride 0.9%
☐ E water for injection

11 Which ONE of the following statements is true regarding the initial dosing and duration of liposomal amphotericin therapy?

☐ A An initial single dose of 150 mg should be administered
☐ B The initial dose must be given over at least 2 hours
☐ C A cumulative dose in the range 1–3 g may be needed for treatment
☐ D Doses higher than 5 mg/kg have a lower propensity for adverse effects
☐ E Treatment duration is limited to 3 consecutive days of therapy

**12** During the infusion, Mrs Y complains of mild muscle and back pain. Which ONE of the following is the most appropriate method of action?

☐ A The infusion should be completed at a faster rate
☐ B The infusion should be continued at a slower rate
☐ C IV chlorphenamine should be administered
☐ D IV paracetamol should be administered
☐ E The infusion should be stopped and a new drug started

Questions 13 and 14 concern Mr SW, a 56-year-old man with diabetes of Caucasian origin who weighs 80 kg and has just been admitted to hospital. He normally takes aspirin, metformin, gliclazide and atorvastatin.

**13** You are reviewing the following blood results as part of your daily ward round with the medical team:

| LABORATORY RESULTS (U&Es) | | | |
|---|---|---|---|
| Sodium | 142 | [135–145] | mmol/L |
| Potassium | 4.6 | [3.5–5.0] | mmol/L |
| Urea | 8.6 | [2.5–7.5] | mmol/L |
| Creatinine | 275 | [60–110] | micromol/L |
| eGFR | 30 | [>90] | mL/min/1.73 $m^2$ |

Select the single most appropriate action in relation to these results.

☐ A Add in a potassium infusion to ensure potassium balance
☐ B Review the need for metformin due to poor tissue perfusion
☐ C Stop gliclazide because it is renally metabolised and will accumulate
☐ D Stop atorvastatin as it is cautioned in renal impairment
☐ E Stop all medication as Mr SW is in end-stage renal failure

**14** Mr SW is suspected of having community-acquired pneumonia and is started on a combination of oral amoxicillin and clarithromycin. Select the ONE interaction that needs your immediate attention from the table below:

| | Drug 1 | Drug 2 | Interaction |
|---|---|---|---|
| A | Aspirin | Gliclazide | Competitive protein binding |
| B | Amoxicillin | Aspirin | Reduced renal clearance |
| C | Amoxicillin | Clarithromycin | Pharmacodynamic antagonism |
| D | Clarithromycin | Atorvastatin | Changes in drug concentration |
| E | Clarithromycin | Gliclazide | Competitive protein binding |

Questions 15–17 concern Mrs A, a 57-year-old postmenopausal woman who suffers from osteopenia. A recent bone density scan confirmed that Mrs A will need to start on alendronic acid 70 mg tablets.

**15** Select the most appropriate biochemical test required prior to treatment initiation.

☐ A albumin level
☐ B magnesium level
☐ C potassium level
☐ D serum calcium level
☐ E sodium level

**16** Select the most appropriate check-up required before treatment is initiated.

☐ A abdominal ultrasound
☐ B chest X-ray
☐ C dental examination
☐ D eye examination
☐ E hip X-ray

**17** Select the single most appropriate piece of counselling advice to provide Mrs A.

☐ A She must take the tablets every day
☐ B She must take the tablets with food
☐ C She must take the tablets while lying down
☐ D She must report any heartburn she experiences
☐ E She need not report any fever on initiation

Question 18 concerns the following extract taken from the BNF regarding the administration of IV ciclosporin:

> ► With intravenous use For *intravenous infusion* (*Sandimmun®*), give intermittently *or* continously *in* Glucose 5% *or* Sodium Chloride 0.9%; dilute to a concentration of 50 mg in 20–100 mL; give intermittent infusion over 2–6 hours; not to be used with PVC equipment. Observe patient for signs of anaphylaxis for at least 30 minutes after starting infusion and at frequent intervals thereafter.

**18** Choose the ONE option that best describes how to administer this product from the table below:

| | **Diluent** | **Infusion concentration** | **Administration set** |
|---|---|---|---|
| A | Glucose 5% | 2.5 mg/mL | PVC |
| B | Glucose 5% | 1 mg/mL | Glass |
| C | Glucose 10% | 0.5 mg/mL | Glass |
| D | Sodium chloride 0.9% | 5 mg/mL | PVC |
| E | Sodium chloride 0.9% | 3.5 mg/mL | Glass |

Questions 19 and 20 concern Child D, a 14-year-old male, who presents with his mother to your chemist with a prescription written by his GP for pain relief following a recent adeno-tonsillectomy procedure in hospital to help relieve sleep apnoea. An extract from the prescription is shown below:

> Codeine Phosphate 25 mg/5 ml Oral Solution
> 6–12 ml QDS PRN for 14/7 days
> Mitte 150 ml

19 Select the ONE option that best describes how you should approach this prescription.

- ☐ A Make a supply as you have no concern over the prescription
- ☐ B Make a supply but provide a 3-day course as per MHRA advice
- ☐ C Refer the patient back to his GP as the product is unsafe for Child D
- ☐ D Refer the patient back to his GP as the duration needs to be changed
- ☐ E Refer the patient back to his GP as the dose of codeine is incorrect

20 With respect to dispensing of codeine in general, what advice would you NOT provide to a patient prescribed this drug at a dose of '30–60 mg QDS PRN'?

- ☐ A To start at a low dose and increase as per GP advice only if your pain is uncontrolled
- ☐ B To take the medication when required for pain relief and use for the shortest time
- ☐ C To continue taking the medication as needed and increase fluid intake if constipation occurs
- ☐ D To continue taking the medication as needed even if it causes drowsiness as this is common
- ☐ E To continue taking the medication even if you have any difficulty in breathing

Question 21 concerns Mr W, a 56-year-old male weighing 55 kg, who presents to the emergency department of your local hospital with right calf pain over the last few days. Urgent blood tests show Mr W to have a significantly raised D-dimer level with impaired liver function.

21 Select the ONE statement that is NOT true regarding the above findings.

- ☐ A A positive D-dimer result indicates that the body contains a high level of cross-linked fibrin by-products
- ☐ B A positive D-dimer result suggests that Mr W may have developed deep vein thrombosis
- ☐ C A positive D-dimer result will necessitate the use of a prophylactic low-molecular-weight heparin product
- ☐ D Depending on the clinical and drug history, unexplained calf pain may be indicative of deep vein thrombosis
- ☐ E An impairment of liver function with respect to prothrombin may be indicative of a problem in the coagulation cascade

Questions 22 and 23 concern Mr TS, a 43-year-old male who takes warfarin for atrial fibrillation. At his most recent anticoagulation clinic appointment, Mr TS was found to have an INR of 3.5. Mr TS explained how he has had a course of antibiotics for a chest infection recently and is due to go to France for 1 week in a few days' time.

22 Which ONE of the following statements best describes Mr TS's presenting condition and subsequent management?

- ☐ A  Mr TS is at risk of bleeding as his INR is lower than normal
- ☐ B  Mr TS's blood is not clotting as quickly as it should be
- ☐ C  Mr TS's antibiotic medication has led to a low INR compared with target
- ☐ D  Mr TS's warfarin dose does not need adjusting to rectify the change in INR
- ☐ E  Mr TS's INR has increased due to a reduction in the effect of warfarin

23 A few days later Mr TS has recovered well and is discharged. Which ONE of the following pieces of advice should he NOT receive?

- ☐ A  Mr TS should be advised to adapt to a Mediterranean diet while on holiday
- ☐ B  Mr TS should be advised to continue his medication as prescribed
- ☐ C  Mr TS should carry his yellow warfarin card and book on him at all times
- ☐ D  Mr TS should not purchase any medication without seeking appropriate advice
- ☐ E  Mr TS should be advised to report any bruising or bleeding to a medical professional

Question 24 concerns the following prescription that you receive from Miss KL while working as a community pharmacist. Miss KL is 26 years old and is due to go for a 2-week holiday to Africa next week.

**Dr A Small**
**Astonbury Medical Centre**
**Birmingham**

**Please supply: Miss KL of 14 Westbury Road, Any Town, A12 4TN**

**Malarone 100/250 mg tablets**

Take 1 tablet daily, starting 2 days before travel and continue for 3 weeks.

Please supply 24 tablets.

| **Signed:** | **GMC Number:** | **Date:** |
|---|---|---|
| A Small | 2671520 | 16/04/16 |

24 Assuming the dose is correct, select the ONE correct statement from those listed below.

- ☐ A You should contact Dr Small as anti-malarial tablets are not allowed on the NHS
- ☐ B You do not need to check if Miss KL is pregnant since malarone is safe in this state
- ☐ C Miss KL should be advised to wear short length clothing while on holiday
- ☐ D A record must be kept in a suitable register if this medication is supplied
- ☐ E This prescription must be sent to the prescription pricing division on month end

Questions 25–27 concern Mrs BH, a 48-year-old female with a PMH of COPD, CCF and glaucoma, who presents to your community pharmacy complaining of a persistent dry cough at night that has not cleared following a recent bout of pneumonia for which she was hospitalised. You check her PMR, which shows that she is on:

| PATIENT MEDICATION RECORD | |
|---|---|
| Seretide 250 Evohaler | **2 puffs BD** |
| Salbutamol 200 mcg Accuhaler | **2 puffs PRN** |
| Ipratropium 20 mcg inhaler | **2 puffs TDS** |
| Latanoprost 0.05% eye drops | **1 drop RE ON** |
| Prednisolone 5 mg tablets | **10 mg ALT DIE** |
| Ramipril 5 mg capsules | **5 mg ON** |
| Furosemide 40 mg tablets | **40 mg OM, 40 mg 2 pm** |
| Senna 7.5 mg tablets | **15 mg ON** |

**25** She tells you that she is unable to sleep at night due to the cough. Select the single most appropriate action that you should take.

- ☐ A Advise Mrs BH to use her salbutamol Accuhaler 20 minutes before going to bed
- ☐ B Advise Mrs BH to purchase a night-time dry cough mixture to help her sleep
- ☐ C Advise Mrs BH to purchase an antihistamine tablet to take before she goes to sleep
- ☐ D Advise Mrs BH to see her GP so he or she can review her medication
- ☐ E Advise Mrs BH that this is normal following a chest infection due to ongoing inflammatory processes

**26** Mrs BH's regular GP calls you for some advice. He tells you that for a few days now she has had a swollen ankle.
Select the single most appropriate advice that you should provide.

- ☐ A You should advise that he increase the 2 pm dose of furosemide to 80 mg
- ☐ B You should advise that he change the prednisolone dosing to 10 mg daily
- ☐ C You should advise that he supply Mrs BH with appropriate compression hosiery
- ☐ D You should advise that he tells Mrs BH to elevate the affected leg daily
- ☐ E You should advise that he asks Mrs BH to reduce her fluid intake for a few days

27 You decide to conduct a medication review on Mrs BH.
Which ONE of the following combinations of drugs has the greatest propensity to cause hypokalaemia?

- ☐ A furosemide, ramipril and senna
- ☐ B ipratropium, *Seretide* and senna
- ☐ C latanoprost, ramipril and senna
- ☐ D prednisolone, salbutamol and furosemide
- ☐ E ramipril, salbutamol and *Seretide*

Questions 28–30 concern the prevention and treatment of venous thromboembolism (VTE).

28 Select the most appropriate time-frame, as suggested by national guidelines, in which a VTE risk assessment must be undertaken in a hospital setting following admission.

- ☐ A 24 hours
- ☐ B 48 hours
- ☐ C 72 hours
- ☐ D 5 days
- ☐ E 1 week

29 Select the ONE risk factor that does NOT increase the risk of VTE.

- ☐ A Active cancer that is currently being treated
- ☐ B Age over 60 years or 35 years if pregnant
- ☐ C Body mass index over 30 $kg/m^2$
- ☐ D Clinically significant dehydration
- ☐ E Family history of cardiac disease

30 The NICE pathway for reducing the risk of VTE is shown below.

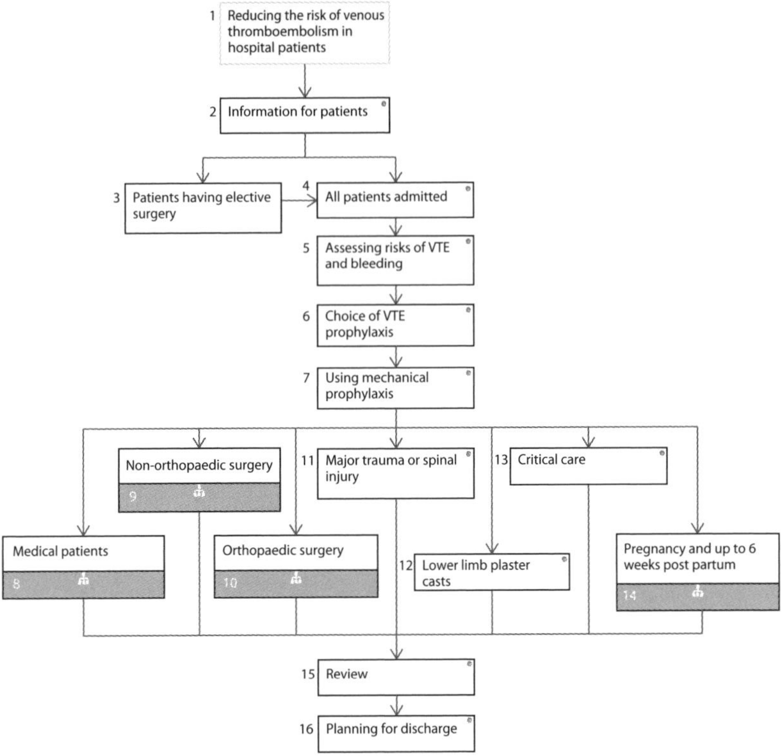


Source: NICE, http://pathways.nice.org.uk/pathways/venous-thromboembolism/reducing-the-risk-of-venous-thromboembolism-in-hospital-patients.pdf

Choose the single most appropriate statement that does NOT correctly explain the pathway.

- ☐ A The pathway applies to hospital patients only
- ☐ B The pathway consists of 16 distinct sections
- ☐ C Within the pathway are four associated sub-pathways
- ☐ D All admitted patients should receive information on VTE
- ☐ E Mechanical prophylaxis refers to the use of walking aids

# *Extended matching questions*

## SECTION A

Ryan Hamilton

In this section, for each numbered question, select the one lettered option that most closely corresponds to the answer. Within each group of questions each lettered option may be used once, more than once or not at all.

**Antibacterials**

- A ciprofloxacin
- B co-amoxiclav
- C co-trimoxazole
- D doxycycline
- E erythromycin
- F flucloxacillin
- G metronidazole
- H nitrofurantoin

For questions 1–5

For the patients described, select the single most likely antibacterial agent from the list above. Each option may be used once, more than once or not at all.

1 Mrs P comes into your pharmacy with a prescription for a short course of an antibacterial to treat cellulitis. Upon looking at her PMR, you note she is currently taking simvastatin 40 mg at night and aspirin 75 mg in the morning. You are worried about a potential interaction between her current medicines and the newly prescribed antibiotic, and advise her to not take the simvastatin during this treatment.

2 Miss J comes into your pharmacy with a prescription for her 8-year-old son Hugh, who has just been prescribed a short course of antibiotics. He is not on any other medicines but you are concerned about the use of this drug in a child of Hugh's age and how it might impact on his development. You decide to ring the prescriber to discuss the treatment.

3 Mr V is a new patient on your care of the elderly ward and has been initiated on a bacterial prophylaxis regimen. While contributing to Mr V's care you note he is also taking spironolactone and bisoprolol. Even though his U&Es are currently in range, you discuss the need for more regular potassium and sodium monitoring because of this newly initiated antibacterial.

4 Mr A is being discharged from your medical assessment unit after being diagnosed with amoebic dysentery. On clerking it was noted that Mr A drinks around 15 units of alcohol per week and you decide to discuss the implications of this in relation to his newly prescribed antibacterial and analgesia medicines.

5 Mrs W is an 83-year-old woman who has just been admitted to the orthopaedic ward after suffering a fall. On further investigation, her fall was not caused by hypotension or dizziness, but by rupture of her Achilles tendon. While taking her medication history you find she has recently taken a course of antibiotics, which you suspect may have contributed to her current condition.

**Antidepressants**

A amitriptyline
B citalopram
C duloxetine
D flupentixol
E mirtazapine
F moclobemide
G St John's wort
H venlafaxine

For questions 6–9

For the patients described, select the single most likely antidepressant from the list above. Each option may be used once, more than once or not at all.

6 Miss K is a 32-year-old woman on your ward and has a long-standing history of depression related to her chronic illness. She has tried antidepressants in the past but stopped them when she felt better. The medical team tell you that she returns to hospital periodically with relapsed symptoms because she stops taking her medicines. They want to treat her depression but the agent they suggest would not be suitable for Miss K considering her non-adherence.

7 One of the new GPs in the surgery across the road calls you for some advice. He has a patient with him, Mr B, who is 28 years old and has agreed to try an antidepressant medicine. Mr B is otherwise fit and healthy, but the GP would like your advice on what to prescribe for this new diagnosis of moderate depression.

8 Three months later you get another call from the GP regarding Mr B, who has not responded well to the initial antidepressants and may be experiencing a number of side-effects. They want to switch him onto a different agent quickly, if not immediately. You inform the GP that one of the drugs he asked about cannot be started immediately.

9 Mrs C has just been admitted onto your emergency admissions unit after being referred directly from her GP, whom she went to see about her headache. On admission she also complains of palpitations and her BP is 205/100 mmHg. Upon taking her history you note she is Japanese and still eats a traditional diet, leading you to suspect her antidepressant medicine may have precipitated this condition.

## Oncology

A bortezomib
B capecitabine
C cyclophosphamide
D doxorubicin
E fluorouracil
F mesna
G mitomycin
H vincristine

For questions 10 and 11

For the patients described, select the single most likely chemotherapy agent from the list above. Each option may be used once, more than once or not at all.

10 You receive a call from one of the nurses, John, working on the chemotherapy day unit about the administration of a medicine to one of his patients. He has never seen this medicine prescribed intrathecally before and wants your advice on how to put up the infusion. You tell him this drug is lethal if given intrathecally and ask to speak to the prescriber.

11 You are clinically reviewing the chemotherapy regimen for Mrs U, who is due to receive her second chemotherapy cycle. While reading her clinical notes you see she complained of blood in the urine, which was diagnosed as haemorrhagic cystitis. When you look at her prescribed chemotherapy you note she has not been prescribed a drug to prevent this side-effect from occurring so you suggest it to the oncologist on the ward.

**Hypercholesterolaemia**

- A atorvastatin
- B colestyramine
- C ezetimibe
- D fenofibrate
- E nicotinic acid
- F *Omacor* (omega-3-acid ethyl esters)
- G orlistat
- H simvastatin

For questions 12–15

For the patients described, select the single most likely medicine from the list above. Each option may be used once, more than once or not at all.

12 Mr M comes into your pharmacy with a prescription for a new medicine to help reduce his cholesterol. After clinically checking the prescription you decide to talk to Mr M about when to take this new medicine, as it is important he takes his other medicines at least 1 hour before or 4–6 hours after taking this new medicine.

**13** You have joined the consultant round on the diabetic ward and the next patient to be seen is Mrs Y, a 46-year-old woman with type 2 diabetes mellitus. Before admission Mrs Y was taking a statin to help reduce her cholesterol, which is at an acceptable level, but during the ward round her triglycerides are found to be 3.1 mmol/L. The medical team ask for your advice on what to prescribe.

**14** Mr Z is a 65-year-old man on your coronary care unit. The medical team have commenced the standard amiodarone initiation regimen but also want to treat his hypercholesterolaemia in light of his cardiac risk. The junior doctor approaches you for advice on what the most appropriate first-line agent would be.

**15** You are a pharmacist working in a GP surgery when Neha, one of the GPs, comes to ask you for some advice about her patient, Mrs A. Mrs A has come in complaining of muscle cramps and pains while taking a statin. This is the second statin Mrs A has tried, so Neha asks you which agent they should try next.

**Vitamins**

- A alfacalcidol (1$\alpha$-hydroxy vitamin $D_3$)
- B alpha-tocopherol (vitamin E)
- C ascorbic acid (vitamin C)
- D cholecalciferol (vitamin $D_3$)
- E hydroxocobalamin (vitamin $B_{12}$)
- F phytomenadione (vitamin $K_1$)
- G thiamine (vitamin $B_1$)
- H retinol (vitamin A)

For questions 16–19

For the patients described, select the single most likely vitamin from the list above. Each option may be used once, more than once or not at all.

**16** Mr E is a man on your general medical ward who is known to have chronic renal disease. While looking through the notes you see his creatinine clearance is currently 21 mL/minute and his adjusted calcium levels are low. You speak to the doctor and both agree to give Mr E a supplement to aid calcium absorption.

17 Miss S, a 23-year-old woman, has just undergone total gastrectomy after being diagnosed with a gastric adenocarcinoma. You note a vital vitamin supplement has not been prescribed and approach the gastroenterology registrar to prescribe this.

18 Miss U comes into your community pharmacy for some advice. She has just found out she is pregnant and would like to improve her diet and take some multivitamins. During your discussion you tell her about a certain vitamin she should avoid taking during pregnancy.

19 Mr O is undergoing active treatment for alcohol misuse and has been receiving *Pabrinex* injections to manage his Wernicke's encephalopathy. His GP would like to convert him to an oral agent and asks your advice on which vitamin to prescribe for this.

**Vaccines, antisera and immunoglobulins**

---

**Vaccines and HIV infection**

HIV-positive individuals with or without symptoms can receive the following live vaccines:

> MMR (but avoid if immunity significantly impaired), varicella-zoster vaccine against chickenpox (but avoid if immunity significantly impaired – consult product literature), rotavirus;

and the following inactivated vaccines:

> anthrax, cholera (oral), diphtheria, *Haemophilus influenzae* type b, hepatitis A, hepatitis B, human papillomavirus, influenza (injection), meningococcal, pertussis, pneumococcal, poliomyelitis, rabies, tetanus, tick-borne encephalitis, typhoid (injection).

HIV-positive individuals should not receive:

> BCG, influenza nasal spray (unless stable HIV infection and receiving antiretroviral therapy), typhoid (oral), yellow fever.

---

Note: The above advice differs from that for other immunocompromised patients; *Immunisation Guidelines for HIV-infected Adults* issued by British HIV Association (BHIVA) is available at www.bhiva.org, and *Immunisation of HIV-infected Children* issued by Children's HIV Association (CHIVA) is available at www.chiva.org.uk

Source: BNF

A *Fendrix* (hepatitis B vaccine)
B *Fluarix Tetra* (influenza vaccine)
C *Fluenz Tetra* (influenza vaccine)
D *Gardasil* (HPV vaccine)
E *Human Rabies Immunoglobulin* (rabies immunoglobulin)
F *Human Tetanus Immunoglobulin* (tetanus immunoglobulin)
G *Menitorix* (haemophilus and neisseria vaccine)
H *MMRvaxPro* (MMR vaccine)
I *NeisVac-C* (meningitis C vaccine)
J *Rhophylac* (anti-D immunoglobulin)

For questions 20 and 21

For the patients described, select the single most likely product from the list above. Each option may be used once, more than once or not at all.

20 Mrs M comes into your pharmacy to collect her monthly supply of *Truvada* (emtricitabine and tenofovir) and asks to speak to you while it is being dispensed. She wants some more information about the routine vaccinations for her 2-month-old daughter who is well and not undergoing any current treatment or receiving any medicines. During your discussion you advise that Mrs M's daughter should avoid receiving a specific product.

21 You are working as the on-call pharmacist for your hospital and are called by one of the A&E doctors, Rumana, who has just received a young man onto the unit who has suffered a stab wound. The patient is unable to confirm his vaccination status and Rumana would like to confirm which product to administer.

**Responding to symptoms in the pharmacy**

A Supply *Dioralyte* with appropriate advice
B Supply lactulose with appropriate advice
C Supply loperamide with appropriate advice
D Supply mebeverine with appropriate advice
E Supply omeprazole with appropriate advice
F Supply *Gaviscon Advance* suspension with appropriate advice
G Supply senna with appropriate advice
H No treatment needed currently, give appropriate advice
I Refer the patient to their GP
J Refer the patient to A&E

For questions 22–27

For the patients described, select the single most appropriate course of action from the list above. Each option may be used once, more than once or not at all.

22 Mr G comes into your community pharmacy complaining of indigestion that has got worse over the last few days. During your discussion, you diagnose him with dyspepsia and find that he is not taking any other medicines, could have a better diet but has lost weight recently without trying.

23 Mr Y comes into your pharmacy this afternoon with his 18-month-old son Jamal, who has been having diarrhoea since yesterday morning. He had five loose, watery motions yesterday and another two this morning. His diet has not changed recently and he does not seem distressed or have a temperature, but he does have slightly dry lips.

24 Mr I asks you for some advice. He has been feeling bloated and having symptoms of mild heartburn and dyspepsia, which started last night after eating some spicy food. He is otherwise well and is not taking any medicines.

25 Miss S comes into your pharmacy looking for something to relieve her constipation. She normally goes once a day but hasn't been for the past 2 days. Whilst she is keen to sort this problem she doesn't claim to be bloated or in pain.

26 Mrs K is looking confused while looking at the 'digestive health' section and you approach her to offer some help. She has been suffering from constipation and hasn't been to the toilet for around 10 days. This has been the first chance to get into the pharmacy. She takes paracetamol for shoulder pain, which she has had for a number of months, but is not experiencing any stomach pains.

27 Miss O is 31 weeks' pregnant and has been experiencing worsening acid reflux, especially at night, which was previously alleviated by using an extra pillow. She has been taking folate-enriched multivitamins during the pregnancy.

**Counselling**

- A Disperse this medicine in a glass of water and take at least 1 hour before bed
- B Do not use sunbeds and protect the skin from sunlight, even on a cloudy day, when taking this medicine
- C Take this medicine as you go to bed and remain lying down for as long as possible
- D Take this medicine at least 30 minutes before food
- E Take this medicine at least 30 minutes before breakfast with a full glass of water, remaining upright for 30 minutes after
- F Take this medicine at least 1 hour before food or other medicines, or 2 hours after
- G Take this medicine with food or just after a meal
- H This medicine can be sucked or chewed before being swallowed

For questions 28–30

For the patients described, select the single most appropriate piece of counselling advice from the list above. Each option may be used once, more than once or not at all.

28 Mrs J has just been to the musculoskeletal clinic for a review of her osteoarthritis and has now been prescribed alendronic acid 70 mg once weekly. As well as advising her to take the medicine on the same day each week you also give her some advice on how best to take the alendronate.

29 Mr Q comes into your community pharmacy with a prescription for his 11-year-old daughter, Olivia, who has acid dyspepsia. She has been prescribed lansoprazole capsules 15 mg daily and her father asks for some advice on how to take them.

30 Miss J presents you with a prescription for flucloxacillin 250 mg QDS for 7 days. When discussing the need to complete the prescribed course you also give her some additional advice on how to take the medicine.

## SECTION B

Babir Malik

In this section, for each numbered question, select the one lettered option that most closely corresponds to the answer. Within each group of questions each lettered option may be used once, more than once or not at all.

### Glaucoma

A acetazolamide
B apraclonidine
C brimonidine
D brinzolamide
E dorzolamide
F latanoprost
G pilocarpine
H timolol

For the scenarios described, select the single most likely eye preparation from the list above. Each option may be used once, more than once or not at all.

1 In 2013, the pH of a branded preparation was reduced from 6.7 to 6.0 to allow for long-term storage at room temperature. Following this reformulation, there has been an increase in the number of reports of eye irritation from across the European Union. The Drug Safety Update (July 2015) advises patients to tell their health professional promptly (within a week) if they have eye irritation (e.g. excessive watering) severe enough to make them consider stopping treatment.
What is the generic name of the brand?

2 Mrs H is 74 years old, has osteoporosis and uncontrolled heart failure.
Which of the above should be avoided?

3 Mr P is 65 years old and has asthma. He is complaining that his eyelashes have become darker, thicker and longer. Mr P thinks it could be due to one of his eye drops.
Which eye drop is most likely the cause?

4 You are explaining about glaucoma to your trainee technician and tell him that there is one preparation that is taken orally as an adjunct to other treatment.
Which of the above is an oral medication?

5 Mr J is a 53-year-old lorry driver who works nights.
Which preparation should be avoided?

**Inhalers**

A aclidinium
B ciclesonide
C glycopyrronium
D indacaterol
E olodaterol
F salbutamol
G terbutaline
H umeclidinium

You are a pharmacist prescriber running a respiratory clinic. You are showing patients a variety of inhalers and asking them which device they prefer, and then choosing a suitable long-acting beta agonist (LABA) or long-acting muscarinic antagonist (LAMA).

For questions 6–10

For the patients described, select the single most likely drug from the list above. Each option may be used once, more than once or not at all.

6 Mr P, a 67-year-old man, likes the *Breezhaler*. He needs a LABA.

7 Mrs, a 42-year-old woman, likes the *Respimat*. She needs a LABA.

8 Mr T, a 32-year-old man, likes the *Genuair*. He needs a LAMA.

9 Miss S, a 30-year-old woman, likes the *Breezhaler*. She needs a LAMA.

10 Mr B, a 19-year-old man, likes the *Ellipta*. He needs a LAMA.

**Contraceptives**

A *Cerazette* (desogestrel)
B *Depo-Provera* (medroxyprogesterone acetate)
C *ellaOne* (ulipristal acetate)
D *Levonelle* (levonorgestrel)
E *Microgynon* (ethinylestradiol with levonorgestrel)
F *Noriday* (norethisterone)
G *Qlaira* (estradiol valerate with dienogest)
H *Zoely* (estradiol with nomegestrol acetate)

For questions 11–15

For the patients described, select the single most likely contraceptive from the list above. Each option may be used once, more than once or not at all.

**11** Miss E, a 23-year-old female, forgets to take her pill every day and would like a long-acting reversible contraceptive.

**12** Mrs C, a 39-year-old female, wants emergency hormonal contraception. She had unprotected intercourse 75 hours ago.

**13** Miss W, a 19-year-old female, is on *Micronor* but doesn't always remember to take it at the same time of day. On occasions, she remembers after 4 hours. She wants to remain on a progesterone-only pill.

**14** Miss G wants an everyday phasic preparation as she forgets to start a new pack after taking a break, and would like different levels of hormones throughout the month because she has been getting too many side-effects.

**15** Mrs B who wants an everyday monophasic preparation as she forgets to start a new pack after taking a break. She was on *Ovranette*.

**Laxatives**

- A bisacodyl
- B dantron
- C ispaghula husk
- D lactulose
- E linaclotide
- F liquid paraffin
- G macrogols
- H senna

For questions 16–20

For the patients described, select the single most likely laxative from the list above. Each option may be used once, more than once or not at all.

16 Miss T is 19 years old and has severe IBS with constipation.
What is the most suitable option?

17 Mr S is terminally ill and constipated.
Which laxative is licensed for use only in terminally ill patients?

18 Mr M is experiencing anal seepage from one of the preparations that he bought from the independent pharmacy while on holiday in Cornwall. Which of the above preparations is he most probably referring to?

19 Mr C needs a laxative that can also be used for hepatic encephalopathy. His GP would like you to recommend a suitable laxative.

20 Mrs B is 30 years old and 26 weeks' pregnant with her second child. She needs a laxative as dietary and lifestyle measures have not helped.

**Antidiabetic medication**

- A *Byetta* (exenatide)
- B *Galvus* (vildagliptin)
- C *Invokana* (canagliflozin)
- D *Lantus* (insulin glargine)
- E *Lyxumia* (lixisenatide)
- F *Starlix* (nateglinide)
- G tolbutamide
- H *Tresiba* (insulin degludec)

For questions 21–25

For the questions below, select the single most likely antidiabetic medication from the list above. Each option may be used once, more than once or not at all.

21 You are undertaking a medication review with Mr D.
Which of the above medicines has a maximum dose of 180 mg TDS?

22 You are asked by a local GP to recommend a drug that is licensed for triple therapy with metformin and a sulfonylurea.

23 Mr H, a 78-year-old man, is on glibenclamide and regularly suffers with hypoglycaemia. You decide to recommend a short-acting sulfonylurea to his GP instead.

24 Mr G comes into your pharmacy and says that the pharmacy across the road gave him the wrong product. He gives you his repeat slip and medication. His repeat slip says 100 units/mL but he has been dispensed 200 units/mL of this product.

25 Mr S has developed a urinary tract infection since starting this medication.

**Substance misuse**

A acamprosate
B buprenorphine
C bupropion
D disulfiram
E lofexidine
F methadone
G nalmefene
H varenicline

For questions 26–30

For the questions below, select the single most likely medication from the list above. Each option may be used once, more than once or not at all.

**26** Mr E has been taking this for 7 weeks and abstinence has not been achieved. You recommend to his GP to discontinue it.

**27** Mr Y asks if he can use his alcohol-containing mouthwash with this preparation and the answer is no.
Which is the most likely medication?

**28** Mr R's alcohol consumption is 65 g per day. He has a high drinking risk level without physical withdrawal symptoms and does not need immediate detoxification. He continues to have a high drinking risk level 2 weeks after initial assessment.
Alongside continuous psychosocial support focused on treatment adherence and reducing alcohol consumption, what should be prescribed according to NICE?

**29** Mr B is suffering from symptoms of opioid withdrawal. You are a senior pharmacist in hospital. The F1 doctor asks you what can be recommended for him.

**30** Miss T is being prescribed this drug but tells you she has started to feel very sad lately since starting this medication.

**Nicotine replacement therapy**

A 3
B 6
C 15
D 16
E 20
F 30
G 40
H 64

You run a smoking cessation service and see four clients today.

For questions 31–35

For the questions below, select the single most likely number from the list above. Each option may be used once, more than once or not at all.

**31** Miss E is using the *Nicorette* nasal spray and wants to know the maximum number of sprays recommended daily?

32 Mrs J asks for how many minutes does one piece of *Nicotinell* chewing gum last.

33 Mr F asks how many minutes a single *Nicorette* 15 mg inhalator cartridge lasts if used intensely.

34 Dr P wants to know the maximum number of *Nicorette Microtabs* recommended daily.

35 Mr F also asks how many minutes a single *Nicorette* 10 mg inhalator cartridge lasts if used intensely.

OTC doses

A 20 mg
B 43.75 mg
C 150 mg
D 500 mg
E 750 mg
F 1200 mg
G 4000 mg
H 4200 mg

You are providing a training session for your counter assistants. What is the maximum daily dose of the following OTC preparations?

For questions 36–40

For the questions below, select the single most likely answer from the list above. Each option may be used once, more than once or not at all.

36 naproxen

37 *Pepto-Bismol*

38 ranitidine

39 ibuprofen

40 flurbiprofen

## SECTION C

Oksana Pyzik

In this section, for each numbered question, select the one lettered option that most closely corresponds to the answer. Within each group of questions each lettered option may be used once, more than once or not at all.

**Ophthalmology**

- A antazoline sulfate 0.5%, xylometazoline hydrochloride 0.05% eye drops
- B chloramphenicol 0.5% eye drops
- C carmellose sodium 0.5% eye drops
- D hypromellose 0.1% eye drops
- E ganciclovir 0.15% gel
- F sodium cromoglicate eye drops
- G timolol 0.25% eye drops
- H tropicamide 0.5% eye drops

For questions 1–5

For the patients described, select the single most likely drug that should be used for the presenting condition. Each option may be used once, more than once or not at all.

1 A 49-year-old man undergoing an examination of the fundus of the eye.

2 A 65-year-old woman who has controlled heart failure and primary open-angle glaucoma.

3 A 6-year-old child who presents with generalised and diffuse redness of the eye, along with mucopurulent discharge in both eyes.

4 A 39-year-old man infected with the herpes simplex virus and presenting with dendritic corneal ulcers.

5 A 26-year-old woman who is pregnant suffers from seasonal allergies which most often affect both her eyes. She is looking for a product that may be used prophylactically to prevent the redness and itching.

**Infectious childhood conditions**

- A chickenpox
- B rubella
- C glandular fever
- D impetigo
- E measles
- F meningitis
- G mollscum contagiosum
- H mumps

For questions 6–10

For the patients described, select which is the most likely infectious childhood condition in each case. Each option may be used once, more than once or not at all.

6 A 16-year-old male patient who presents with swollen glands, fever, malaise and headache as well as a maculopapular rash that appears on the trunk.

7 A 12-year-old child who presents with Koplik's spots and a rash that first appears on ears and face, and then progresses to trunk and limbs.

8 A 4-year-old child who presents with fever, lethargy, stiff neck, vomiting, photophobia and a rash with purplish blotches.

9 A 10-year-old child who presents with a rash on the facial area concentrated around the nose and mouth, with vesicles that exude yellow forming crusts.

10 A 9-year-old boy who presents with several small and localised lesions with yellow exudate. The injuries were sustained while playing sport. He was subsequently prescribed topical fusidic acid.

**Gastrointestinal**

A bisacodyl
B colestyramine
C docusate sodium
D lactulose
E liquid paraffin
F macrogols
G omeprazole
H prucalopride

For questions 11–16

For the patients described, select which drug is most appropriate in each case. Each option may be used once, more than once or not at all.

**11** A 53-year-old woman with chronic constipation who has tried stimulant, osmotic and bulk-forming laxatives, which have failed to provide an adequate response.

**12** A 23-year-old man who is suffering from diarrhoea associated with Crohn's disease.

**13** A 6-year-old child suffering from severe constipation that has not been resolved by diet alone.

**14** A 50-year-old man who presents with alarm symptoms and has a family history of colorectal cancer. He will be undergoing a colonoscopy procedure for further investigation.

**15** A 42-year-old woman who is seeking the fastest-acting medicine to treat her acute constipation.

**16** A 55-year-old man who has a confirmed case of *Helicobacter pylori* infection and has also been prescribed the following medicines:

Amoxicillin 500 mg three times daily
Metronidazole 400 mg three times daily

**Monitoring high-risk and commonly prescribed medicines**

A amiodarone
B aspirin
C digoxin
D lithium
E methotrexate
F phenytoin
G theophylline
H warfarin

For questions 17–21

For the patients described, select the most appropriate drug in each case. Each option may be used once, more than once or not at all.

17 A 43-year-old man who has just suffered a myocardial infarction with ST-segment elevation, and has been treated with oxygen and slow IV injection of diamorphine to manage pain. He requires reperfusion therapy. Which medicine is most likely to be given for this medical emergency?

18 A 52-year-old man has had a recent change in medication during his last hospital visit. He must undergo a chest X-ray, and liver function and thyroid function tests before initiating the new treatment and then followed up every 6 months. The patient requires a loading dose of 200 mg TDS for 7 days, then 200 mg BD for 7 days, followed by a maintenance dose of 200 mg once daily.

19 A 76-year-old woman suffers from moderate rheumatoid arthritis and is monitored every 2–3 months for blood dyscrasias and liver cirrhosis.

20 A 50-year-old man has been prescribed 200 mg tablets BD and has his plasma concentrations measured 5 days after starting the oral treatment and at least 3 days after any dose adjustment. He is also taking tiotropium; however, his treatment with ciprofloxacin has been discontinued.

21 The doctor on your ward has switched Mrs P, a 62-year-old woman, from the IV to the oral route of her medicine for heart failure. As a result the dose must be increased by 20–33% to maintain the same plasma concentration of the drug.
Which of the above medicines has the doctor prescribed?

**Adverse effects**

- A hyperuricaemia
- B hypocalcaemia
- C hyperkalaemia
- D hypokalaemia
- E hypermagnesaemia
- F hypomagnesaemia
- G hypernatraemia
- H hyponatraemia

For questions 22–26

For the patients described, select the most appropriate adverse effect. Each option may be used once, more than once or not at all.

22 Mrs B is a 59-year-old woman who has been prescribed allopurinol, alongside her cancer chemotherapy treatment, to prevent which imbalance?

23 Mr X is a 61-year-old man suffering from hypertension. He has been taking bendroflumethiazide 2.5 mg tablets daily. However, his liver function has rapidly declined and he is at risk of hepatic failure. This electrolyte imbalance may precipitate encephalopathy.

24 Miss J is a 52-year-old woman who has been prescribed a thiazide diuretic as an adjunct to her current antihypertensive treatment to achieve better control of her blood pressure. Her potassium levels are normal and her records show she has alcoholic cirrhosis of the liver. She has developed arrhythmia as a result of this electrolyte imbalance.

25 A 46-year-old man has been prescribed ciclosporin for severe acute ulcerative colitis and is also taking ramipril 10 mg daily for hypertension. You identify that the above interaction may precipitate this electrolyte imbalance.

26 A 24-year-old male has been prescribed lithium for the treatment and prophylaxis of bipolar disorder. He presents at hospital with benign intracranial hypertension, persistent headache and visual disturbance, polyuria and polydipsia. This electrolyte imbalance may worsen symptoms.

**Pathogens causing disease**

A *Aspergillus niger*
B *Chlamydia psittaci*
C *Escherichia coli*
D *Legionella pneumophila*
E *Staphylococcus aureus*
F *Streptococcus pneumoniae*
G *Trichomonas vaginalis*
H *Pseudomonas aeruginosa*

For questions 27–31

For the patients described, select the pathogen most likely to be the cause of the infection for each disease state. Each option may be used once, more than once or not at all.

27 Mr C has suffered from recurring infection of the right outer ear and has received prolonged antibiotic treatment. He has presented to the GP with fungal overgrowth in his right ear and was subsequently diagnosed with otomycosis. This pathogen is the most likely cause of the infection.

28 Miss M presents with profuse, frothy, greenish-yellow and malodorous discharge accompanied by vulvar itching and dysuria. This pathogen is the most likely cause of the infection.

29 Mr B is a breeder of birds and has travelled the world to buy wild parrots. Two weeks after returning from his travels he has developed severe pneumonia accompanied by splenomegaly. Blood analysis shows leukopenia, thrombocytopenia and moderately elevated liver enzymes. This pathogen is the most likely cause of the infection.

30 Mr P is an 82-year-old man who has just returned from a cruise to Mexico. He particularly enjoyed the hot tub and pool facilities on the ship. One week after his return he developed an uncommon form of severe community-acquired pneumonia accompanied by chest pain and mental confusion. This pathogen is the most likely cause of the infection.

31 Mrs R is a 61-year-old woman who has developed hospital-acquired pneumonia. She is being treated with piperacillin with tazobactam by intravenous infusion 4.5 g every 8 hours. This pathogen is the most likely cause of the infection.

**Parasiticidal preparations**

A dimeticone
B fipronil
C ivermectin
D malathion
E mebendazole
F praziquantel and pyrantel embonate
G selenium sulfide
H zinc pyrithione

For questions 32–37

For the patients described, select the most appropriate drug for each case. Each option may be used once, more than once or not at all.

32 Mr G presents with a severe case of Norwegian scabies in which hyperkeratotic, warty crusts have developed. This medicine has been prescribed at a dose of 200 mcg/kg.

33 A mother describes her 5-year-old child's symptoms as including peri-anal itching which is worse at night. This medicine is taken as a single dose.

34 This is an organophosphorus insecticide that is used as an alternative for the treatment of head lice. Resistance may be an issue with this product.

35 This is effective against *Pediculus humanus capitis* and acts on the surface of the organism.

36 This may be used as a lotion and left on the affected area for 10 minutes before rinsing off. It should be applied once daily for 7 days, and the course repeated if necessary. It is used to treat pityriasis (tinea) versicolor.

37 Mr U is looking for an appropriate medicine to deworm his cat named Jinxy. This medicine is effective against *Toxocara cati*.

**Topical preparations**

A amorolfine
B salicylic acid and lactic acid
C glutaraldehyde
D formaldehyde
E terbinafine
F silver nitrate
G miconazole
H mupirocin

For questions 38–40

For the patients described, select the most appropriate drug for each case. Each option may be used once, more than once or not at all.

38 Mr H presents with tinea unguium of his toenails. You advise him to apply this medicine to the infected nails once or twice a week following filing and cleansing. He should allow the nail to dry for about 3 minutes and review treatment every 3 months.

39 Miss Q presents at your pharmacy with concerns about unsightly raised bumps on her index finger. You recommend a medical product and advise that it may cause chemical burns on surrounding skin, and may stain skin and fabric. In addition, you advise her to remove dead skin by gentle filing before use and then to cover with an adhesive dressing after application.

40 Miss Y is a nurse at the local care home and has been confirmed as a carrier of nasal meticillin-resistant *Staphylococcus aureus* (MRSA). This medicine is to be applied 2–3 times daily to the inner surface of each nostril.

## SECTION D

Amar Iqbal

In this section, for each numbered question, select the one lettered option that most closely corresponds to the answer. Within each group of questions each lettered option may be used once, more than once or not at all.

### Cardiovascular

A aspirin
B amiodarone
C amlodipine
D bumetanide
E chlorothiazide
F digoxin
G eplerenone
H furosemide

For questions 1–4, select the most appropriate drug choice or drug culprit in each of the following clinical situations.

1 Mr HF, a 56-year-old man, presents to hospital with oedema secondary to worsening left ventricular dysfunction. Mr HF's weight has increased by 5 kg in the last 3 days and the doctors suspect resistance to his furosemide treatment. A more potent drug of the same class is required.

2 Mr IR, a 63-year-old man with atrial fibrillation, is noticed to have a resting pulse of 56 bpm by the nurse taking his observations in the morning. The nurse consults the duty doctor who requests that she does not administer his regular cardiac glycoside today due to this finding.

3 Mr DM, a 46-year-old man with diabetes, presents to the emergency department following persistent blood glucose levels greater than 20 mmol/L as well as joint pain and swelling. Blood results show a plasma urate level that is three times normal. He tells you that he has recently started a new drug to control his blood pressure.

4 Mrs AF, a 53-year-old woman who is on regular treatment for atrial fibrillation, presents to your chemist complaining of muscle pain that she has not experienced before. She was discharged from the hospital last month on simvastatin 40 mg daily.

**Prescription charges and record retention**

A 0
B 1
C 2
D 3
E 4
F 5
G 6
H 7

For questions 5–9 choose the one option that correctly correlates to either the number of NHS prescription charges or the number of years for which a particular record must be retained in the accompanying scenarios.

5 The duration in years for which the responsible pharmacist records must be kept once fully completed.

6 The number of charges levied against a prescription for hydroxycarbamide 500 mg capsules and ondansetron 4 mg tablets supplied to a 53-year-old man suffering from chronic myeloid leukaemia.

7 The number of charges levied against a prescription for one pair of class 1 below-knee compression stockings supplied to a pregnant woman for varicose veins.

8 The number of charges a prescription for omeprazole 20 mg tablets, amoxicillin 500 mg capsules, metronidazole 400 mg tablets and *Fortisip* (strawberry and vanilla flavours) will carry when supplied to a 38-year-old male being treated as an inpatient in hospital for disease-related malnutrition secondary to a perforated ulcer.

9 The number of years for which a controlled drug register entry must be kept following the final entry and issue of a new register.

**Cautionary and advisory labels**

- A Warning: This medicine may make you sleepy. If this happens, do not drive or use tools or machines. Do not drink alcohol
- B Warning: Do not drink alcohol
- C Warning. Do not stop taking this medicine unless your doctor tells you to stop
- D Warning: Read the additional information given to you with this medicine
- E This medicine may colour your urine. This is harmless
- F Take 30–60 minutes before food
- G Do not take indigestion remedies 2 hours before or after you take this medicine
- H Take with a full glass of water

Which of the above recommended cautionary and advisory wording applies in the scenario(s) described below?

10 A 23-year-old man is discharged from hospital with dapsone 100 mg tablets, which he is taking to treat *Pneumocystis jirovecii* pneumonia.

11 A 14-year-old boy is discharged from hospital with flucloxacillin 500 mg capsules, which he must take for 2 weeks in order to completely treat cellulitis.

12 A 46-year-old male is discharged from hospital with metronidazole 400 mg tablets for a further 5 days as prophylaxis against infection following an abdominal procedure.

13 A 6-year-old boy is written a prescription by his GP for nitrofurantoin 25 mg/mL suspension as prophylaxis for recurrent urinary tract infections.

**Neurology**

- A carbamazepine
- B diazepam
- C levetiracetam
- D lorazepam
- E midazolam
- F phenobarbital
- G phenytoin
- H sodium valproate

For questions 14–16, select the ONE option from above that correctly corresponds to the product described in the given situation(s):

14 Child M, a 3 year old with epilepsy who is on your ward, has a seizure. The seizure continues for over 5 minutes. The doctor asks for your advice as to which product is suitable and that he can give via the buccal route as the child does not have any IV access port.

15 Mrs W, a 33-year-old female, presents to your chemist with a prescription for her regular anti-epileptic medication. You do not have her specific brand (*Keppra*) in stock and decide to provide a generic product. What is the name of the generic drug that you supply?

16 Child S, a 5-year-old child, presents to hospital with his mother. You are ascertaining a medication history from his mother who tells you that he is maintained on a twice-daily dose of his regular anti-epileptic medication but she is unable to remember the name. She tells you that her GP prescribes a special alcohol-free and sugar-free preparation because the licensed product contains 38% alcohol. She also has to sign the back of a prescription form when she collects it from her community pharmacy. Which product is Child S most likely to be on?

**Cardiovascular**

- A aspirin
- B atorvastatin
- C bisoprolol
- D glyceryl trinitrate
- E oxygen
- F prasugrel
- G ramipril
- H simvastatin

For questions 17–20, select the ONE drug from the above options that applies in the given situation(s).

17 You are running a cardiac workshop for patients who are currently under the care of your hospital with unstable angina. Mr R, a 55-year-old man, asks you what he should do if he gets central chest pain radiating to the left-hand side of his body.
Which drug should he be advised to chew on while arranging for an ambulance?

**18** Mr D, a 66-year-old man who is admitted to the admission unit of your hospital, is diagnosed as having a non-ST-elevated myocardial infarction (NSTEMI).
Which drug should he be prescribed prior to percutaneous coronary intervention?

**19** Mr F, a 63-year-old man, presents to your community pharmacy asking for some advice on relieving symptoms of angina. He asks you if he is able to purchase a drug for 'relieving chest pain' over the counter from you.
Which drug can Mr F theoretically buy to help control this symptom of his condition?

**20** Mrs G, a 55-year-old woman, is due to be discharged from hospital following an NSTEMI.
Which of the above is the drug of first choice in preventing secondary cardiovascular complications following an NSTEMI?

**Adverse drug reactions**

A Stop taking the drug and report to your GP or local hospital immediately
B Stop taking the drug and make a routine appointment with your GP
C Continue taking the drug and speak with your GP to change to an alternative
D Continue taking the drug as normal since this reaction is harmless
E Continue taking this drug as normal and report the reaction to your GP
F Report this to the MHRA even though this product/device is not intensively monitored
G Report this reaction to the MHRA as this product/device is intensively monitored
H Report this error to the MHRA via a yellow card report

For questions 21–23, select which ONE of the above pieces of advice best matches that which you would provide in each of the following scenarios.

**21** A 56-year-old male admitted to hospital with a fall due to severe hypotension since starting dapagliflozin tablets (▼) 3 days ago.

**22** A 23-year-old woman who presents to your chemist complaining of facial flushing due to her *Tensipine* (nifedipine) MR tablets, after her GP increased the dose yesterday.

23 A 35-year-old man who complains to you that the 'flu vaccine' he had yesterday has caused him to come out in a rash all over his body.

**Central nervous system**

A 10 mg TDS
B 20 mg TDS
C 50 mg TDS
D 100 mg TDS
E 120 mg TDS
F 200 mg TDS
G 300 mg TDS
H 400 mg TDS

For questions 24–27, select the most appropriate dose for the product as detailed in the given situation(s) below:

24 The dose of metoclopramide that should be prescribed for a 24-year-old female who has presented the second time in a fortnight with hyperemesis.

25 The dose of cyclizine that should be prescribed PRN for a 33-year-old female who requires it post-surgery to prevent nausea and vomiting.

26 The standard dose of orlistat that should be prescribed before a meal for a 36-year-old female as an adjunct in the management of obesity.

27 The initial dose of gabapentin that should be prescribed for a 42-year-old male to treat neuropathic pain.

**Over-the-counter scenarios**

A Advise initially to increase fluid intake
B Advise the purchase of paracetamol
C Advise the purchase of some throat lozenges
D Advise the purchase of some loperamide
E Advise the purchase of an eye ointment
F Advise that no treatment is necessary
G Advise waiting for 2 days and then seeing the GP
H Advise seeking urgent medical attention

For questions 28–30, choose the ONE best piece of advice you should provide as a pharmacist in each of the following situations.

28 Mr JS asks for your advice as he has recently been bruising easily and seems to be coming down with a 'sore throat and flu'. You check his PMR and note he recently started carbimazole 5 mg tablets.

29 Mrs WP asks for your advice on her 2-month-old son who has been quite irritable recently and has now had two episodes of diarrhoea in the last 24 hours.

30 Mr DW enquires as to whether he can purchase some ibuprofen for some muscle and joint pain, which occurred as a result of some heavy gardening. He tells you he normally takes sertraline.

**Nutrition and blood**

A hypocalcaemia
B hypercalcaemia
C hypokalaemia
D hyperkalaemia
E hypomagnesaemia
F hyponatraemia
G hypophosphataemia
H hyperphosphataemia

For questions 31–33, select the ONE best option that closely matches the electrolyte imbalance in the clinical situation(s) described below:

31 Mrs SW, a 33-year-old female, is admitted to hospital with nausea, vomiting, muscle weakness and increasing confusion over the last 3 days. Her medication history consists of citalopram 20 mg once daily.

32 Mr TS, a 46-year-old male, is admitted to the intensive care unit with a history of fatigue, muscle spasms and nystagmus. He has been on omeprazole 20 mg once daily for the past year.

33 Mrs FM, a 66-year-old male, has been recently started on a one-off intravenous infusion of pamidronate based on consistent serum blood results, which showed a particularly severe electrolyte imbalance.

**Respiratory**

A inhaled beclomethasone
B inhaled salbutamol
C IV aminophylline
D IV hydrocortisone
E nebulised ipratropium
F oral montelukast
G oral prednisolone
H oral theophylline

For questions 34–36, select the ONE best option that should be utilised or trialled next in each of the clinical situations described below:

34 Child F, a 14-year-old male with uncontrolled asthma for the past 6 weeks, who presents to your asthma clinic and already has a 'preventer' and 'reliever'.

35 Child S, a 7-year-old female who has presented with acute severe asthma who requires an anti-inflammatory agent but is unable to swallow.

36 Mr W, a 34-year-old male who is on *Slo-phyllin* capsules as well as regular maximum dose inhaled therapy, who has been admitted to hospital four times in the last 3 months due to persistent poor symptom control.

**Diabetes**

A diazoxide
B gliclazide
C glucagon
D glucose 50% infusion
E insulin infusion
F *Lantus Solostar* pen
G *Lucozade* energy drink (55 mL)
H metformin

For questions 37–40, select the product of choice in each of the clinical situations described below:

37 Mr R, a 43-year-old male who is a known diabetic, tells you that he has been feeling confused and dizzy, and his heart is beating faster this morning. You advise him to check his blood glucose levels, but if needed which of the above products should be administered?

38 You are taking a drug history from Mrs W, a 56-year-old female who tells you she has been recently started on a new medication for her diabetes due to having poor renal function. She is unsure of its name and asks you if you know. You check her PMR and find her to be on one of the above products.
Which drug is Mrs W most likely to have been started on?

39 Child H, a 10-day-old neonate, is suffering from intractable hypoglycaemia that has not been controlled using standard treatment. It is decided to start him on oral therapy using an agent based on its side-effect profile.
Which agent is most likely to be utilised?

40 Mr TS, a 26-year-old man newly diagnosed with type 2 diabetes mellitus, is to be initiated on treatment to help control his blood glucose levels as his diet has failed to help control this.
Which drug should Mr TS be started on?

# Calculation questions

## SECTION A

### Ryan Hamilton

Questions 1–4 concern Bhavesh, an 11-year-old boy on your children's surgery unit. The nutrition team saw him this morning and wrote the following prescription for TPN:

| | |
|---|---|
| **Name:** PATEL, Bhavesh | **Ward:** CSU |
| **DOB:** 05/06/2005 | **Day of TPN:** 1–2 |
| **NHS:** 123 456 0000 | **Number of bags:** 2 |
| | **Duration/bag:** 24 hours |
| **Weight:** 28.6 kg | |
| **Height:** 135 cm | **Infusion rate:** |
| **Volume:** 1044 mL | **Calcium:** 26.0 mmol |
| | **Iron:** nil |
| **Total energy:** 1800 kcal | **Magnesium:** 14.3 mmol |
| **Glucose:** 900 kcal | **Phosphate:** 28.6 mmol |
| **SMOF Lipid:** 900 kcal | **Potassium:** 41.5 mmol |
| | **Sodium:** 57.2 mmol |
| **Solvito:** 1 mL | |
| **Vitilipid:** 10 mL | **Peditrace:** 28.5 mL |
| **Prescriber:** *Dr Smith* | **Pharmacist:** *J Jones* |
| **Date:** 02/02/2016 | **Date:** 02/02/2016 |

Your aseptic unit has the following table of molecular masses for the compounds commonly used to make up TPN:

| Formula | g/mol | Formula | g/mol | Formula | g/mol |
|---|---|---|---|---|---|
| $CaCl_2$ | 110.88 | $K_2HPO_4$ | 174.18 | NaCl | 58.44 |
| $CaCl_2{\cdot}2H_2O$ | 147.01 | $MgC_3H_7PO_6$ | 194.4 | $NaO_2C_2H_2$ | 82.03 |
| KCl | 74.55 | $MgCl_2$ | 95.21 | $C_6H_{12}O_6$ | 180.16 |

1 How many millilitres of calcium chloride dihydrate solution 13.4% w/v will you need to get the necessary calcium requirements for the above TPN regimen? Give your answer to one decimal place.

2 Your aseptic suite stocks potassium chloride solution 15% w/v for TPN. How many 10-mL ampoules will be needed to make up this TPN regimen? Give your answer in whole ampoules.

3 At what rate should the TPN be infused (mL/hour)? Give your answer to one decimal place.

4 The medical team call you about the above TPN regimen. They are reviewing the patient and may need to fluid restrict him. They ask you how much fluid the patient is getting per kilogram of body weight. Give your answer as a whole number.

5 One of the nurses calls you from the neonatal intensive care unit regarding starter parenteral nutrition for one of her patients. Earlier in the day your pharmacy department supplied the ward with a 50-mL vial of glucose 50% and a 500-mL bag of glucose 20%. The nurse needs to make up a 50-mL syringe containing 30% glucose. What volume of glucose 50% will the nurse need to use? Give your answer to one decimal place.

6 Mrs Q is a 71-year-old patient on your stroke unit who has a compromised swallow and is not tolerating a nasogastric tube. Before admission she was taking one co-beneldopa 12.5/50 mg capsule four times a day and one co-beneldopa 25/100 mg MR capsule at night for Parkinson's disease. The medical team are worried about this medicine being omitted as it will impede recovery, so they ask you to convert her to a rotigotine patch.

**Guide for estimating equivalent levodopa dosages for rotigotine patches.[6]**

1. Calculate Adjusted Levodopa Equivalent Daily Dose (LEDD):

[(A) + (B)] x 0.55 = ______mg

**(A) Total adjusted daily levodopa dose**

Total daily levodopa dose in mg (excluding benserazide or carbidopa)
[eg Madopar 125mg QDS = 4x100=400mg/24h]
X 0.7 (if MR/CR preparation) **or**
X 1.3 (if on COMT inhibitor) **or**
X 0.91 (if MR/CR preparation and on COMT inhibitor)
= ______mg

**(B) Total adjusted daily dopamine agonist estimate levodopa equivalent dose**

Total daily dopamine agonist in mg
X 100 (if on pramipexole/cabergoline/pergolide)
X 20 (if on ropinirole/rotigotine)
X 10 (if on apomorphine/bromocriptine)
= _____mg

(the above figures refer to each medication's levodopa equivalent factor)

(continue overleaf)

NB (A) or (B) = 0 if not taking that type of medication

2. Calculate dosage for rotigotine patch = Adjusted LEDD /20 = ____mg

- Round to nearest 2mg (to max of 16mg) and prescribe as 24-hour patch.
- DO NOT cut patches – available as 2mg/4mg/6mg/8mg patches (can use more than one patch).
- Treat each patient individually and adjust doses accordingly:
  - if increased stiffness/slowness observed, increase dose and review daily
  - if increased confusion/hallucinations observed, decrease dose and review daily
- If adjusted LEDD >350mg, use rotigotine 16mg and consult with specialist regarding administration of apomorphine.

12 13 14

Source: Parkinson's UK, Emergency treatment of patients with Parkinson's, http://www.parkinsons.org.uk/sites/default/files/publications/download/english/pk0135_emergencymanagement.pdf

Using the Parkinson's UK resource given above, what strength of rotigotine patch should Mrs Q be prescribed?

Questions 7–9 concern the prescribing and administration of aminophylline infusions. The following is an extract from an aminophylline prescribing proforma, which can be used to support your calculations.

| **NHS Trust**<br><br>**Aminophylline Infusion Proforma** | **Actual body weight: __________kg**<br><br>Aminophylline does not distribute into fatty tissue. Ideal body weight needs to be used for obese patients<br>**Male: 50 kg + 2.3 kg for every inch over 5 ft**<br><br>**Female: 45.5 kg + 2.3 kg for every inch over 5 ft** | [Attach Patient Label] |
|---|---|---|

| **Intravenous Loading Dose = 5 mg/kg over 20 minutes** | | |
|---|---|---|
| **Intravenous** | Elderly/heart failure | 0.3 mg/kg/hr |
| **Maintenance Dose** | Non-smoking Adult | 0.5 mg/kg/hr |
| As continuous infusion<br>Rates in mL/hr | Smoking Adult | 0.7 mg/kg/hr |

Source: Adapted from University Hospitals of Leicester NHS Trust's aminophylline proforma

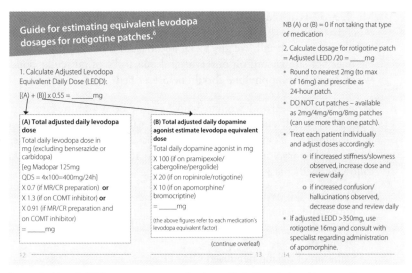

7 Mr J, a 32-year-old man, has been admitted to ITU with a severe exacerbation of asthma and needs to be initiated on aminophylline. He is 6 feet 1 inch tall, weighs 82 kg and has no other co-morbidities. He does not smoke and on observation looks to be of muscular build. What dose of aminophylline should be prescribed?

8 Mrs D is a 75-year-old woman who has just been admitted to your respiratory ward with an exacerbation of asthma. On admission she was weighed at 97 kg and states her height as 5 feet 3 inches. When taking her history you find she quit smoking 10 years ago and is on the following medicines:

*Fostair* 100/6 two puffs BD
Budesonide 4 mg PO OM
*Phyllocontin Continus* (aminophylline) 225 mg tablets, two tablets BD MDU
Salbutamol 2.5 mg nebulised QDS PRN
Salbutamol 100 mcg CFC-free inhaler 2–6 puffs QDS PRN via an aerochamber (blue)

How much aminophylline should Mrs D receive over the next 24 hours? Give your answer to the nearest whole number.

9 Miss B, a 24-year-old woman, has been prescribed a post-loading aminophylline infusion to run for 24 hours. Her height is 5 feet 3 inches and she was weighed as 52 kg. She has been unable to quit smoking and it is likely that this exacerbated her asthma. The nurses have made up aminophylline 500 mg in 500 mL glucose 5% and ask you at what rate to set the infusion pump. Give your answer to one decimal place.

10 You are on the ward round with the medical team and they want to prescribe meropenem for one of their patients, Mr F. His serum creatinine is 134 μmol/L and his eGFR has been reported as 32 mL/minute/1.73 $m^2$ through the laboratory results system. You note that he is 83 years old and weighs only 54 kg.
You decide to calculate his renal function using the Cockcroft–Gault formula. Give your answer to one decimal place.

For question 11 you can use the SPC for dimethyl fumarate to support your calculations: http://www.medicines.org.uk/emc/medicine/28593

11 Mr Y comes into your pharmacy with a new prescription from his GP who is a specialist in dermatology. The prescriber has written the following:

*Dimethyl fumarate 120 mg PO MDU as per standard initiation regimen. Supply 4/52.*

How many dimethyl fumarate 120 mg tablets will you need to supply to cover the prescribed course?

12 Mrs B comes into your pharmacy with a prescription for her 12-year-old daughter, who has been prescribed flucloxacillin 125 mg/5 mL suspension at a dose of 125 mg QDS for 7 days.
Given that, when 100 mL of the suspension is made up it has an expiry date of 7 days, how many bottles should you supply?

Questions 13 and 14 concern the stratified prescribing of digoxin for cardiac patients based upon pharmacokinetic principles. The following equations may need to be used to support your calculations:

$$\text{Non-heart failure DigCl (L/hour)} = (0.06 \times \text{CrCl (mL/minute)}) + (0.05 \times \text{IBW (kg)})$$

$$\text{Heart failure DigCl (L/hour)} = (0.053 \times \text{CrCl (mL/minute)}) + (0.02 \times \text{IBW (kg)})$$

$$C_{pss} = \frac{(F \times D)}{(\text{DigCl} \times t)}$$

Male IBW = 50 kg + 2.3 kg for every inch over 5 feet
Female IBW = 45.5 kg + 2.3 kg for every inch over 5 feet

13 Mrs Z is a 67-year-old woman who requires rapid digitalisation but has not responded to the first dose of digoxin. Out of curiosity you decide to estimate the rate at which she is clearing the digoxin doses. You obtain the following observations from her notes:

| | | |
|---|---|---|
| **Weight:** 95 kg | **Height:** 5′4″ | **Age:** 67 years |
| **HR:** 82 BPM | **BP:** 130/90 | **Temp:** 37°C |
| **Creatinine:** 84 μmol/L | **$K^+$:** 4.0 mmol/L | **Urea:** 5.1 mmol/L |

Calculate Mrs Z's estimated digoxin clearance to two decimal places.

14 Mr E is suffering from heart failure. On medical review he has responded well to the IV loading dose of digoxin and the medical team want to place him on long-term oral therapy, aiming for a serum digoxin of 2.0 mcg/L (acceptable range 1.5–2.0 mcg/L). You glean the following information from his notes:

| | | |
|---|---|---|
| **Weight:** 75 kg | **Height:** 6′0″ | **Age:** 74 years |
| **HR:** 71 BPM | **BP:** 143/95 | **Temp:** 37°C |
| **Creatinine:** 153 µmol/L | **$K^+$:** 3.4 mmol/L | **Urea:** 6.1 mmol/L |

Calculate the daily dose that Mr E should initially be prescribed. Note digoxin tablets come in 62.5 mcg, 125 mcg and 250 mcg strengths and are only 63% bioavailable.

15 Mrs G attends your respiratory clinic for a review of her COPD, which seems to have worsened over the past 6 months. She is currently taking salbutamol PRN and you are considering stepping up her treatment. In order to prescribe the optimal therapy, you decide to measure her $FEV_1$, which you find to be 1.39 L/s.
Calculate Mrs G's $FEV_1$ as a percentage of her predicted normal value (2.10 L/s). Give your answer to the nearest whole number.

Questions 16–18 concern the supply and administration of intravenous immunoglobulin (IVIG). You extract the following information from the national Department of Health guidance and the SPC:

| **Product** | **Infusion rates** | | **Infusion time of 70 g in minutes at max. rate** |
|---|---|---|---|
| | **Initial** | **Maximum** | |
| **Baxter Kiovig** | 0.5 mL/kg/h for 30 min | 6 mL/kg/h (8 ml/kg/h in PID) | 100 |
| **BPL Gammaplex** | 0.01–0.02 mL/kg/min for 15 min | 0.04–0.08 mL/kg/min | 250 |
| **BPL Vigam** | 0.01–0.02 mL/kg/min for 30 min | 0.04 mL/kg/min (max. 3 mL/min) | 500 |
| **Biotest Intratect** | 1.4 mL/kg/h for 30 min | 1.9 mL/kg/h | 640 |

Source: Clinical guidelines for immunoglobulin use, second edition update, Department of Health (2011)

16 Krishna is a 9-year-old girl on a paediatric HDU who has been admitted with acute immune thrombocytopenic purpura and requires IVIG at a dose of 0.8 g/kg, which can be repeated at a later date if she does not respond.
Given that Krishna weighs 28 kg and your hospital stocks *Intratect* (IV human immunoglobulin) 5 g (100 mL) and 10 g (200 mL) vials, how much IVIG should you supply for the initial infusion? Give your answer in grams as per the products available.

**17** When the *Intratect* gets to the ward, the nurses ask you how long Krishna's treatment will take if they are unable to increase the infusion rate above the initial rate.
Calculate the time taken to infuse the *Intratect* at the slowest advisable rate to the nearest whole number.

**18** If Krishna tolerates the IVIG, the nursing team hope to increase the rate of infusion up to the maximum rate in steps of 0.1 mL/kg per minute every 15 minutes.
Assuming they are able to achieve the fastest rate of infusion, how long will Krishna's treatment take to complete from start to finish? Calculate the time to the nearest whole number.

**19** You have received a prescription for Mr L, a 92-year-old man, who is receiving end-of-life care, is developing swallowing problems and has poor vascular access. His consultant has written a prescription for 14 × 1 g suppositories containing morphine sulfate 5 mg, which she would like you to make up extemporaneously. You find the displacement value of morphine sulfate is 1.6 and you work out a formula to make 16 suppositories.
Calculate how much witepsol you would need. Give your answer to two decimal places.

**20** You have received a prescription for Miss W for 150 g of coal tar and salicylic acid ointment BP, which you have to make up extemporaneously. From the *British Pharmacopoeia* 2015 you obtain the following master formula and method:

| **Extemporaneous Preparation of *Coal Tar and Salicylic Acid 2% w/v in an emulsifying base*** | |
|---|---|
| Coal tar | 20 g |
| Polysorbate 80 | 40 g |
| Salicylic acid | 20 g |
| Emulsifying wax | 114 g |
| White soft paraffin | 190 g |
| Coconut oil | 540 g |
| Liquid paraffin | 76 g |

Source: BP 2015, http://www.pharmacopoeia.co.uk/bp2015/ixbin/bp.cgi?a=display&r=PGDUWidqIU7&n=1206&id=5473&all=yes

Allowing for a 10% excess, how much salicylic acid should be weighed out to fulfil this supply? Give your answer to two decimal places.

21 Mrs F is due to commence a course of chemotherapy and the consultants would like to dose her by BSA. You look at Mrs F's notes and find that she is 1.3 m tall and weighs 73 kg.

$BSA\ (m^2) = ([\text{height (cm)} \times \text{weight (kg)}]/3600)^{0.5}$

Calculate Mrs F's BSA to one decimal place.

22 Mr R has recently been admitted to your ward with delirium and has been refusing his medicines. Before admission he was taking digoxin 125 mcg every morning and so the medical team feel it necessary to administer this parenterally. You discuss the fact that oral digoxin is only 63% bioavailable and an IV dose of 125 mcg is inappropriate. Calculate the equivalent daily IV dose of digoxin to one decimal place.

23 Mrs I, who weighs 62 kg, requires an IV infusion of dopamine hydrochloride, which has been prescribed at a rate of 3 mcg/kg per minute. The nurses have infusion bags of 160 mg dopamine in 100 mL of glucose 5%.
Calculate the rate at which the infusion pump should be set to one decimal place.

24 Mr V has been admitted to your ward and has been prescribed phenytoin capsules 150 mg TDS. He is having swallowing difficulties so you suggest phenytoin liquid, which you know is not bioequivalent; 100 mg of phenytoin sodium is equivalent to 90 mg of the phenytoin base. Calculate how many millilitres of phenytoin suspension 30 mg/5 mL Mr V will need for each dose.

25 Mr K is one of your cystic fibrosis patients and presents you with a prescription for IV flucloxacillin 2 g QDS, to be administered through the local OPAT scheme. Each flucloxacillin 1 g vial is reconstituted in 20 mL water for injections, given over 30 minutes and flushed with 4 mL water for injections before the line is locked.
How many injection ampoules of 10 mL water should be supplied to cover a 2-week course?

Questions 26 and 27 concern the prescribing of paracetamol in children. The following table may be used to support your calculations.

**Pain; pyrexia with discomfort**

- **By mouth**

  Neonate 28–32 weeks' corrected gestational age 20 mg/kg as a single dose then 10–15 mg/kg every 8–12 hours as necessary, max. 30 mg/kg daily in divided doses
  Neonate over 32 weeks' corrected gestatational age 20 mg/kg as a single dose then 10–15 mg/kg every 6–8 hours as necessary, max. 60 mg/kg daily in divided doses
  Child 1–3 months 30–60 mg every 8 hours as necessary, max. 60 mg/kg daily in divided doses
  Child 3–6 months 60 mg every 4–6 hours (max. 4 doses in 24 hours)
  Child 6 months–2 years 120 mg every 4–6 hours (max. 4 doses in 24 hours)
  Child 2–4 years 180 mg every 4–6 hours (max. 4 doses in 24 hours)
  Child 4–6 years 240 mg every 4–6 hours (max. 4 doses in 24 hours)
  Child 6–8 years 240–250 mg every 4–6 hours (max. 4 doses in 24 hours)
  Child 8–10 years 360–375 mg every 4–6 hours (max. 4 doses in 24 hours)
  Child 10–12 years 480–500 mg every 4–6 hours (max. 4 doses in 24 hours)
  Child 12–16 years 480–750 mg every 4–6 hours (max. 4 doses in 24 hours)
  Child 16–18 years 500 mg–1 g every 4–6 hours (max. 4 doses in 24 hours)

- **By rectum**

  Neonate 28–32 weeks' corrected gestational age 20 mg/kg as a single dose then 10–15 mg/kg every 12 hours as necessary, max. 30 mg/kg daily in divided doses
  Neonate over 32 weeks' corrected gestational age 30 mg/kg as a single dose then 15–20 mg/kg every 8 hours as necessary; max. 60 mg/kg daily in divided doses
  Child 1–3 months 30–60 mg every 8 hours as necessary; 60 mg/kg daily in divided doses
  Child 3–12 months 60–125 mg every 4–6 hours as necessary (max. 4 doses in 24 hours)
  Child 1–5 years 125–250 mg every 4–6 hours as necessary (max. 4 doses in 24 hours)

Child 5–12 years 250–500 mg every 4–6 hours as necessary (max. 4 closes in 24 hours)

Child 12–18 years 500 mg every 4–6 hours

- **By intravenous infusion over 15 minutes**

  Preterm neonate over 32 weeks' corrected gestational age 7.5 mg/kg every 8 hours
  Neonate 10 mg/kg every 4–6 hours, max. 30 mg/kg daily
  Child body weight under 10 kg 10 mg/kg every 4–6 hours; max. 30 mg/kg daily
  Child body weight 10–50 kg 15 mg/kg every 4–6 hours, max. 60 mg/kg daily
  Child body weight over 50 kg 1 g every 4–6 hours, max. 4 g daily

---

Source: BNFC

26 Vikki is a 6-year-old girl, weighing 16.4 kg, on your paediatric intensive care unit and the medics want to prescribe IV paracetamol every 6 hours for her.
How much paracetamol should be prescribed for each dose?

27 Aled is a 4-day-old male infant on your neonatal unit who has a suspected infection and has had a temperature spike. He was born approximately 8 weeks early and only weighs 1.14 kg. His team note he looks agitated and want to prescribe the highest dose of regular oral paracetamol they can.
Considering the oral solution is 120 mg/5 mL, how much paracetamol should be prescribed to give a measurable dose? Give your answer to one decimal place.

28 Miss T has been prescribed dexamethasone 13.2 mg IV daily until her condition begins to respond. The injections contain 4 mg dexamethasone phosphate (equivalent to 3.3 mg base) per millilitre.
How many millilitres of this would you advise the nurses to administer for each dose?

29 You are the on-call pharmacist for your hospital and receive a call from one of the nurses about the reconstitution of a high-dose benzylpenicillin IV infusion and whether this should be given peripherally or centrally. The patient has no central access and the highest concentration of benzylpenicillin that can be given peripherally is 600 mg in 10 mL. What is the minimum volume of 0.9% sodium chloride each 2.4 g dose should be dissolved in?

30 What weight of zinc oxide powder must you add to 15 g of 1% (w/w) zinc oxide cream to produce a cream of 3% (w/w)? Give your answer to one decimal place.

31 What concentration of chlorhexidine acetate solution (mg/mL) must be made up so that when 5 mL of this is diluted to 200 mL it gives a chlorhexidine concentration of 0.05%?

32 Dr Harb contacts you regarding a trial he is considering running. He wants to investigate the application of intrathecal acetylcysteine 2% and asks how you might formulate a 10-mL syringe. You know the product will need to be isotonic with the cerebrospinal fluid, of which you find the average freezing point to be −0.5770°C. From your research you learn that you may need to add sodium chloride to the formulation to make it isotonic. You find the freezing point depression value of a 1% sodium chloride solution to be 0.5760°C and find the freezing point depression value of a 1% acetylcysteine solution to be 0.1135°C.

$$W = \frac{f - a}{b}$$

$W$ is the amount (% w/v) of adjusting compound to be added
$f$ is the freezing-point depression of the target body fluid
$a$ is the freezing-point depression of the drug solution(s)
$b$ is the freezing-point depression of a 1% solution of adjusting compound

Calculate how much sodium chloride must be added to make the product isotonic. Give your answer to two decimal places.

33 You are a pharmacist in the R&D team of a specials manufacturing company and are working on a salicylic acid solution that could be used in the ears and eyes. One of your starting points is to estimate the pH of the candidate 1.5% salicylic acid solution. The molar mass of salicylic acid is 138.21 g·mol$^{-1}$ with a p$K_a$ of 2.97 at 25°C.

$$K_a = \frac{[H^+][A^-]}{[HA]}$$

Calculate the estimated pH of this solution to two decimal places.

**34** Mr L is taking digoxin and his serum concentration has just come back from the lab as 3.23 mcg/L. The registrar wants to initiate *DigiFab*. He was weighed on admission as 72 kg.

No. of *DigiFab* vials required

$$= \frac{\text{(patient weight (kg)} \times \text{digoxin level (mcg/L))}}{100}$$

How many whole vials of *DigiFab* should be used to treat Mr L?

**35** Miss R is 28 weeks' pregnant and has been diagnosed with anaemia from iron deficiency. A trial with oral ferrous gluconate has failed to produce a clinically relevant response and the obstetric team now want to trial her on IV *Venofer* to achieve a haemoglobin level of 14 g/dL. Miss R's notes contain the following information:

Age: 23 years
Height: 5 feet 3 inches
Weight before pregnancy: 54 kg
Gestation: 28 weeks
Iron: 4.2 micromol/L
Haemoglobin: 8.6 g/dL
BP: 134/91 mmHg

Calculate the volume of *Venofer* Miss R will need over the course of her treatment. Give your answer to the nearest whole millilitre.
The SPC for *Venofer* can be used to support your calculations: http://www.medicines.org.uk/emc/medicine/24168.

**36** You are a pharmacist working for a generic manufacturer and the current rotary tablet press is able to make 2700 tablets per minute. The company wants to upgrade to a more efficient rotary press and you have found a model that can make up to 4100 tablets per minute. Calculate the percentage increase in yield obtained over a 3-hour run. Give your answer to one decimal place.

**37** Mr J brings in a prescription for *Zomorph* (morphine sulfate modified release) 30 mg capsules and *Zomorph* 60 mg capsules, with a prescribed regimen of 90 mg BD. He has also been prescribed *Oramorph* 10 mg/5 mL oral solution, 2 mg to be taken when needed for pain relief. You believe this dose to be too small and discuss breakthrough pain doses with the GP, who asks you what the usual maximum breakthrough dose of *Oramorph* would be for this patient.
Calculate the maximum breakthrough dose of *Oramorph*.

38 Miss N comes to see you about losing weight and would like some advice. During the consultation you take some weights and measurements and find that she is 1.67 metres tall and weighs 99.6 kg.
How much weight does Miss N need to lose in order to reach a healthy BMI of 24 $kg/m^2$? Give your answer to one decimal place.

39 Mr O has been admitted to your endocrine unit with diabetic ketoacidosis requiring urgent treatment. He has been prescribed 500 mL sodium bicarbonate 1.26% (12.6 g, 150 mmol, per litre) and a short course of *Sandocal* 1000 effervescent tablets (containing 25 mmol calcium and 5.95 mmol sodium) one tablet BD. You inform the medical team to monitor his sodium levels closely.
How much sodium will Mr O be receiving in the next 24 hours? Give your answer to one decimal place.

40 Mr J calls you up to ask for some advice. His 3-month-old son Sam has recently been prescribed long-term oral hydrocortisone 1 mg at 8 am in the morning then 0.5 mg at 12 pm and 4 pm. He has been supplied 10 mg hydrocortisone tablets, which he was advised to crush and disperse, but he is not sure how much to administer. Hydrocortisone tablets are scored so you advise him to disperse half a tablet in 10 mL of water.
How much of this dispersion should be given for the morning dose?

## SECTION B

Babir Malik

Questions 1 and 2 concern Jimmy, a 4-month-old infant weighing 4.7 kg.

BNF dose – 4 mg/kg BD

1 Jimmy has been diagnosed with an acute urinary tract infection, sensitive to trimethoprim.
How much trimethoprim suspension 50 mg/5 mL in mL to one decimal place should be dispensed for a 5-day course in practice?

2 How many mL should Jimmy receive twice daily?

3 You receive the following prescription for Mrs B:

Topiramate 25 mg tablets
Take ONE in the morning for 2 weeks
Then take ONE in the morning and ONE in the evening for 2 weeks
Then take TWO in the morning and ONE in the evening for 2 weeks
Then take TWO in the morning and TWO in the evening for 2 weeks
Then take THREE in the morning and TWO in the evening for 2 weeks
Then take THREE in the morning and THREE in the evening for 4 weeks

How many tablets should be dispensed in total?

4 Concentrated waters, such as rose water, peppermint water and chloroform water, are used to produce single-strength waters. They are intended for dilution in the ratio 1 part concentrated water to 39 parts water. To prepare a double-strength water, we have to take twice the volume of a concentrated water.
A formula requires 276 mL double-strength peppermint water, but you only have the concentrate in stock.
How much concentrate in mL do you need?

5 A lotion contains 26% v/v glycerin.
How many litres of glycerin should be used to prepare 7 L of the lotion?

6 You are asked to prepare a 70-L batch of drug A (0.09% w/v). You have available to you a 68% w/v concentrate.
How much of this concentrate do you need to use, rounded to the nearest 0.1 mL?

7 Miss L, a 26-year-old woman weighing 60 kg and 1.59 m tall, comes into your pharmacy and asks to purchase *Alli*. This can be sold only to patients with a BMI over 28.

BMI = weight (kg)/height (m)$^2$

What is her BMI to one decimal place?

8 Kevin, the local pharmacist prescriber, has prescribed paediatric chloral elixir for a child. You decide to make it up as an extemporaneous preparation.
What quantity of chloral hydrate is there in grams in 183 mL of the elixir?
Formula: chloral hydrate 200 mg, water 0.1 mL, blackcurrant syrup 1 mL, syrup to 5 mL.

9 You are teaching your pre-registration pharmacy technician about suppositories and explaining the displacement value as the number of parts of suppository ingredients that displace 1 gram of the base.
The approximate cocoa butter displacement value for zinc oxide is 5, which means 5 g of this ingredient will displace 1 g of the cocoa butter base.
Calculate the quantity of cocoa butter in grams required to make seven suppositories (3-g mould) each containing 300 mg of zinc oxide.

10 Mr G is a 64-year-old man weighing 77 kg. He has been prescribed IV sodium valporate at a dose of 30 mg/kg over 5 minutes.
Calculate the rate (mL/minute) at which the sodium valporate should be injected. *Epilim* IV 400 mg/4 mL is available on the ward.

11 Sarah, a 3-month-old full-term infant, weighing 5.6 kg, has been prescribed *Augmentin* injection 600 mg (or co-amoxiclav 500/100). She is to be given the dose by IV infusion.
What daily volume in mL will be given assuming that each vial is made up to 10 mL?

12 You mix together 360 g of 5% w/w calamine in white soft paraffin (WSP), 275 g of 1% w/w calamine in WSP and 85 g of WSP.
What is the %w/w concentration of calamine in the mixture to two decimal places?

13 You receive a prescription for adrenaline injection 1 in 40 000 5-mL ampoules × 10.
What is the weight (mg) of adrenaline contained in 5 mL of adrenaline injection 1 in 40 000?

14 Mrs M brings in a prescription for *Timodine* cream on a Saturday afternoon.
*Timodine* cream 30 g contains hydrocortisone 0.5%, nystatin 100 000 units/g, benzalkonium chloride solution 0.2%, dimeticone '350' 10%.
What is the weight in mg of hydrocortisone contained in 30 g of *Timodine* cream?

15 Mr S is directed to use 150 mL of a 1 in 8000 solution of potassium permanganate each day for a week. He is going away on a plane and must not take more than 100 mL of any liquid in his hand luggage. The prescription directs you to make a solution 20 times this strength so that Mr S can dilute it to 1050 mL before use, which will last for one week.
How much potassium permanganate in mg, to two decimal places, will be required to dispense this prescription?

16 Mr M presents a prescription for prednisolone 40 mg a day for 5 days, then reducing by 5 mg every 3 days.
How many tablets would you need to supply for the whole course?

Questions 17 and 18 relate to Mr RW, a 64-year-old plumber. He brings in a prescription for *Ciloxan* drops for his left eye only.

BNF dose:
Day 1: 1 drop every 15 minutes for 6 hours then every 30 minutes
Day 2: 1 drop every hour
Days 3–14: 1 drop every 4 hours

17 Assuming he is able to follow the dosage schedule exactly, how many drops in total should Mr W instil into his left eye?

18 Assume there are 20 drops in 1 mL. *Ciloxan* is available in a 5-mL bottle.
How many bottles would you need to supply to Mr W for the course?

19 Mr JS brings in a prescription for his 6-year-old son Justin for 10 g clobetasol propionate 0.02% cream.
How much clobetasol propionate 0.05% cream in grams would you have to mix in order to fulfil the prescription?

20 A 4-month-old infant of average weight is prescribed drug X for which there is no known paediatric dose. The adult total daily dose is 1200 mg. A 4-month-old child should receive 25% of the adult daily dose. Drug X should be given TDS. Drug X is available as an oral solution containing 50 mg/5 mL.
What dose should the child be given?

## SECTION C

Oksana Pyzik

1 Miss A weighs 65 kg and is given dobutamine by IV infusion at a rate of 2.5 mcg/kg per minute.
What dose of dobutamine (mg) will have been administered after 1 hour?

2 Mr P has been prescribed amitriptyline 25 mg tablets. The prescriber's instructions are shown below:

> Rx Amitriptyline 25 mg tablets
> Sig: 150 mg ON for 5 days then reduce by 25 mg every 5 days then stop

How many tablets will you dispense for Mr P?

3 A child weighing 6.6 kg is prescribed a dose of 12 mg/kg per day of ciprofloxacin, to be given by IV infusion in two divided doses.
What volume of ciprofloxacin infusion 2 mg/mL should be given for each dose. Give your answer to the nearest decimal place.

4 Mr Q, a 52-year-old man, is suffering from the advanced stages of lung cancer and is undergoing palliative care treatment. He is prescribed a diamorphine syringe driver and usually takes oral morphine 180 mg BD to control his pain. The syringe driver contains 15 mL of diamorphine 20 mg/mL.

| **Equivalent doses of morphine sulfate and diamorphine hydrochloride given over 24 hours** | | |
|---|---|---|
| **These equivalences are *approximate only* and should be adjusted according to response** | | |
| MORPHINE | | PARENTERAL DIAMORPHINE |
| Oral morphine sulfate | Subcutaneous infusion of morphine sulfate | Subcutaneous infusion of diamorphine hydrochloride |
| **over 24 hours** | **over 24 hours** | **over 24 hours** |
| 30 mg | 15 mg | 10 mg |
| 60 mg | 30 mg | 20 mg |
| 90 mg | 45 mg | 30 mg |
| 120 mg | 60 mg | 40 mg |
| 180 mg | 90 mg | 60 mg |
| 240 mg | 120 mg | 80 mg |
| 360 mg | 180 mg | 120 mg |
| 480 mg | 240 mg | 160 mg |
| 600 mg | 300 mg | 200 mg |
| 780 mg | 390 mg | 260 mg |
| 960 mg | 480 mg | 320 mg |
| 1200 mg | 600 mg | 400 mg |
| If breakthrough pain occurs give a subcutaneous (preferable) or intramuscular injection equivalent to one-tenth to one-sixth of the total 24-hour subcutaneous infusion dose. It is kinder to give an intermittent bolus injection *subcutaneously* – absorption is smoother so that the risk of adverse effects at peak absorption is avoided (an even better method is to use a subcutaneous butterfly needle). To minimise the risk of infection no individual subcutaneous infusion solution should be used for longer than 24 hours. | | |

What rate should the syringe driver be set at (in mL/hour) so the patient receives the equivalent dose of diamorphine?

5 Mrs L is taking *Morphgesic* SR 70 mg BD for chronic pain in terminal bowel cancer. She has just been started on *Oramorph* for breakthrough pain. According to the BNF, the breakthrough dose is one-tenth to one-sixth of the total daily dose.
What is the appropriate dose volume (mL) as a range of *Oramorph* that Mrs L can safely take?

6 Mr W has been prescribed hydroxyzine hydrochloride syrup 10 mg/5 mL with the following instructions for use:

> Rx:
> Hydroxyzine hydrochloride syrup 10 mg/5 mL
> Initially 15 mg ON for 1/52
> Then 25 mg ON for 1/52
> Then 25 mg BD

What exact volume of hydroxyzine hydrochloride syrup 10 mg/5 mL is required for a 28-day supply?

7 A 3-month-old infant weighing 6 kg has been prescribed folic acid at a dose of 500 mcg/kg per day. The folic acid you have in stock contains 62.5 mg of folic acid per 125 mL.
What volume of syrup should be given daily?

8 Mr G is a 53-year-old man who suffers from follicular non-Hodgkin's lymphoma and has been prescribed rituximab. The consultant rings the pharmacy to ask for a dose based on BSA. You look at Mr G's notes and see that he is 1.5 m tall and weighs 80 kg.
BSA ($m^2$) = [height (cm) × weight (kg)/3600]$^{0.5}$
Calculate Mr G's BSA to one decimal place.

9 Mrs SB has a BSA of 1.5 $m^2$ and has been prescribed fludarabine by mouth at a dose of 40 mg/$m^2$ daily for 5 days. You are asked to dispense a 5-day course of tablets for Mrs SB.
How many 10-mg tablets are required for the 5-day course?

10 Miss Z is admitted to hospital for an overdose of verapamil with a toxic plasma concentration of 74 mcg/mL. The drug's half-life is 8.5 hours.
How long, in hours, will it take for plasma concentration to fall to 2.3125 mcg/mL? Assume absorption and distribution are complete and elimination is described by a first-order reaction.

11 What weight of adrenaline (micrograms) is contained in 1 mL of adrenaline injection 1 in 10 000?

12 Mr M is prescribed an oxygen cylinder (1360 L) and giving set. The prescriber has instructed to set the flow rate at 2 L/minute.
If given continuously, for how long will the cylinder provide treatment?

13 Mrs U is 62 years old and has been diagnosed with Parkinson's disease. She has been initiated on apomorphine injections in hospital. She has been discharged with a supply of 20-mg/2-mL ampoules and U100 insulin 1-mL syringes with needles. She requires a subcutaneous dose of 1.5 mg.
How many units should Mrs U draw up each time when using her syringe?

14 What weight of ingredient is required to produce 1000 mL of a solution such that, when 2.5 mL of it is diluted to 50 mL with water, it gives a 0.25% w/v solution?

15 A coated tablet has a dry weight of coating of 10 mg/tablet. The coating solution is prepared to contain 10% w/v of coating material.
How long is needed to coat a batch of 1 million tablets at a spray rate of 250 mL/minute, given that coating efficiency is 100%?

16 Mr C is receiving a diamorphine infusion over 24 hours. He is currently receiving a dose of 150 mg over a 24-hour period using a syringe pump that is calibrated to 36 mm/24 hours (note that some syringe pumps are calibrated in mm/hour). You increase the rate of infusion to 54 mm/24 hours.
What dosage will the patient receive in 24 hours following the increased rate of infusion?

17 A 6-year-old child who weighs 16 kg is being treated in order to prevent a secondary case of meningococcal meningitis. The consultant seeks your advice as to a suitable dose of rifampicin for the child.
According the BNFC:
'Rifampicin 600 mg every 12 hours for 2 days; child under 1 year 5 mg/kg every 12 hours for 2 days; 1–12 years 10 mg/kg every 12 hours for 2 days.'
What total volume of rifampicin 100 mg/5 mL syrup should be dispensed?

18 You receive a prescription for 2.8% w/w sulfur in aqueous cream. What weight of sulfur do you need to make 175 g?

19 What is the concentration of dextrose in a solution prepared by mixing together 200 mL of 10% w/v dextrose solution, 50 mL of 20% w/v dextrose solution and 150 mL of 5% w/v dextrose solution? Give your answer to one decimal place.

20 Mr F's GP would like to gradually withdraw his corticosteroid treatment. The GP has issued a prescription with the instructions to take 25 mg daily for 1 week. From week 2 onwards, the daily dose should be reduced by 2.5 mg every 7 days.
What is the exact number of prednisolone 2.5-mg tablets that will be required for a 42-day supply?

## SECTION D

Amar Iqbal

1 You are responding to a call from your ward sister for advice on how to make up a 30% glucose solution. Upon checking the stock list you find that the ward keeps the following products:

Glucose 50% injection (10-mL ampoules)
Glucose 10% infusion bag (100 mL)

You advise the ward sister to mix the two products to create 100 mL of the desired 30% solution.
What volume of glucose 50% injection (mL) is required as part of this dilution?

2 You are required to calculate the eGFR of Child M, a 12-year-old boy, who is suspected of having an acute kidney injury secondary to IV gentamicin.
Given that Child M is 6 feet tall, weighs 52 kg and his current serum creatinine is 410 micromol/L, what is his eGFR (mL/minute per 1.73 $m^2$)?

eGFR = 40 × height (cm)/SeCr (micromol/L)

and 1 foot is equivalent to 30 cm

3 You are required to freshly prepare 100 mL of double-strength chloroform water using concentrated chloroform water.
What volume (mL) of concentrated chloroform water is needed to prepare the double-strength chloroform water?

4 Master JW has been stable on *Epanutin Infatabs* at a dose of 50 mg BD for the past 2 months. Following a seizure, his GP is due to increase his dose to 60 mg BD and at the same time switch him over to *Epanutin* suspension 30 mg/5 mL for ease.

**Dose equivalence and conversion**

Preparations containing phenytoin sodium are **not** bioequivalent to those containing phenytoin base (such as *Epanutin Infatabs* and *Epanutin* suspension); 100 mg of phenytoin sodium is approximately equivalent in therapeutic effect to 92 mg phenytoin base. The dose is the same for all phenytoin products when initiating therapy; however, if switching between these products the difference in phenytoin content may be clinically significant. Care is needed when making changes between formulations and plasma-phenytoin concentration monitoring is recommended.

- **MEDICINAL FORMS**
  There can be variation in the licensing of different medicines containing the same drug. Forms available from special-order manufacturers include: oral suspension, oral solution.

  **Tablet**
  CAUTIONARY AND ADVISORY LABELS 8

  ▶ **PHENYTOIN (Non-proprietary)**
  **Phenytoin sodium 100 mg** Phenytoin sodium 100 mg tablets | 28 tablet PoM £117.00 DT price = £30.00

  **Chewable tablet**
  CAUTIONARY AND ADVISORY LABELS 8, 24

  ▶ **Epanutin (Phenytoin)** (Pfizer Ltd)
  **Phenytoin 50 mg** Epanutin Infatabs 50 mg chewable tablets | 200 tablet PoM £13.18

  **Capsule**
  CAUTIONARY AND ADVISORY LABELS 8

  ▶ **PHENYTOIN (Non-proprietary)**
  **Phenytoin sodium 25 mg** Phenytoin sodium 25 mg capsules | 28 capsule PoM £15.74 DT price = £15.74
  **Phenytoin sodium 50 mg** Phenytoin sodium 50 mg capsules | 28 capsule PoM £15.98 DT price = £15.98
  **Phenytoin sodium 100 mg** Phenytoin sodium 100 mg capsules | 84 capsule PoM £50.00–£67.50 DT price = £54.00
  **Phenytoin sodium 300 mg** Phenytoin sodium 300 mg capsules | 28 capsule PoM £57.38 DT price = £57.38

  **Oral suspension**
  CAUTIONARY AND ADVISORY LABELS 8

  ▶ **Epanutin (Phenytoin)** (Pfizer Ltd)
  **Phenytoin 6 mg per 1 ml** Epanutin 30 mg/5 ml oral suspension | 500 ml PoM £4.27 DT price = £4.27

**Solution for injection**

EXCIPIENTS: May contain alcohol, propylene glycol

ELECTROLYTES: May contain sodium

- ▶ **PHENYTOIN (Non-proprietary)**
  **Phenytoin sodium 50 mg per 1 ml** Phenytoin sodium 250 mg/5 ml solution for injection ampoules | 5 ampoule PoM £14.55–£24.40 | 10 ampoule PoM no price available
- ▶ **Epanutin (Phenytoin sodium)** (Pfizer Ltd)
  **Phenytoin sodium 50 mg per 1 ml** Epanutin Ready-Mixed Parenteral 250 mg/5 ml solution for injection ampoules | 10 ampoule PoM £48.79

What volume (mL) of suspension will provide the required 60-mg dose?

5 What mass (g) of beclomethasone diproprionate 1% cream is required to make 100 g of *Betnovate RD* (0.025%) cream?

6 Child M has been prescribed enoxaparin 0.5 unit/kg twice daily for the treatment of a cerebral infarct.
Given that Child M weighs 24 kg, what dose in units will he receive over a 1-week period?

7 You are required to supply prednisolone 5-mg soluble tablets against the following instructions for a 6-year-old child of average height and weight, with a BSA of 0.80 m$^2$, who is being discharged from hospital with nephrotic syndrome:
*60 mg/m$^2$ OM for 1 week, then reduce to 40 mg/m$^2$ for 1 week, then reduce to 20 mg/m$^2$ for 1 week, then reduce to 10 mg/m$^2$ for 1 week until clinic review. Round the dose to the nearest 5 mg at each stage.*
How many prednisolone 5-mg soluble tablets will you dispense until the clinic review?

8 Calculate the volume of solution that is required to fulfil the following prescription with an overage of 8 mL to allow for any losses on transfer.
Ranitidine 75 mg/5 mL oral solution 15 mg TDS for 14 days

9 What volume (mL) of 50% w/v glucose is required to produce 500 mL of 25% w/v glucose?

**10** Mr DW gives you a prescription for 500 g of 0.1% w/w *Dermovate* in *Unguentum Merck* cream.
Calculate the weight (mg) of *Dermovate* needed for this prescription.

**11** Mrs H, a 47-year-old woman weighing 60 kg, is admitted to hospital for a hysterectomy. The surgeon decides to give Mrs H some propofol 1% for induction at a dose of 2.5 mg/kg and a rate of 20 mg every second until response.
Calculate the minimum time period (in seconds) of anaesthesia that Mrs H will receive.

**12** One *Permitab* tablet when diluted with 4 L of water provides a 1 in 10 000 solution.
What is the percentage (%) strength of this solution?

**13** Mrs SW is prescribed some *Gaviscon Advance* suspension to help control her symptoms of reflux.
Approximately how many millimoles of sodium ions are present in 20 mL of this product? [*Gaviscon Advance* suspension contains 2.3 mmol/sodium per 5 mL.]

**14** *Arovit* contains 150 000 units of vitamin A per 30 drops.
How much vitamin A (in units) is present in 12 drops of this mixture?

**15** How many millimoles of potassium chloride concentrate 15% is required to prepare 500 mL of a solution containing 3 mmol/kg per day of potassium ions for a neonate weighing 2 kg with a daily fluid intake of 150 mL/kg per day? Give your answer to the nearest whole number.

**16** What mass (mg) of adrenaline is required to make 500 mL of a 1 in 1000 preparation?

**17** You are required to calculate the amount of dobutamine (mg) that a patient has received while on a continuous infusion. The patient weighs 60 kg and the infusion device was set 12 hours ago at 10 mcg/kg per minute.

**18** Cefotaxime has been prescribed in a child for suspected meningitis. It has a half-life of 6 hours.
If the initial plasma level of cefotaxime is 1 g/L, what is the plasma level (mg/L) of this drug after 18 hours?

**19** A 4-year-old child who weighs 18 kg is admitted to hospital after taking an accidental overdose of paracetamol 250 mg/5 mL suspension. It is decided to start him on an IV infusion of acetylcysteine.
Using the extract below, calculate the volume of diluent (mL) that is needed to dilute the initial dose for this child.

- Neonate: Initially 150 mg/kg over 1 hour, dose to be administered in 3 mL/kg glucose 5%, followed by 50 mg/kg over 4 hours, dose to be administered in 7 mL/kg glucose 5%, then 100 mg/kg over 16 hours, dose to be administered in 14 mL/kg glucose 5%.
- Child (body weight up to 20 kg): Initially 150 mg/kg over 1 hour, dose to be administered in 3 mL/kg glucose 5%, followed by 50 mg/kg over 4 hours, dose to be administered in 7 mL/kg glucose 5%, then 100 mg/kg over 16 hours, dose to be administered in 14 mL/kg glucose 5%
- Child (body weight 20–39 kg): Initially 150 mg/kg over 1 hour, dose to be administered in 100 mL glucose 5%, followed by 50 mg/kg over 4 hours, dose to be administered in 250 mL glucose 5%, then 100 mg/kg over 16 hours, dose to be administered in 500 mL glucose 5%
- Child (body weight 40 kg and above): 150 mg/kg over 1 hour, dose to be administered in 200 mL Glucose Intravenous Infusion 5%, then 50 mg/kg over 4 hours, to be started immediately after completion of first infusion, dose to be administered in 500 mL Glucose Intravenous Infusion 5%, then 100 mg/kg over 16 hours, to be started immediately after completion of second infusion, dose to be administered in 1 litre Glucose Intravenous Infusion 5%

Note: Glucose 5% is preferred infusion fluid; sodium chloride 0.9% is an alternative if glucose 5% unsuitable
Source: BNFC

20 Child S is an immunocompetent 12-year-old boy of average body weight and height who requires IV aciclovir every 8 hours over a period of 5 days for herpes zoster infection.
The BNFC dose for IV aciclovir is 250 mg/m$^2$ every 8 hours for 5 days, and the BSA for a 12 year old is 1.3 m$^2$.
Calculate the volume of aciclovir 25 mg/mL IV infusion required for a single intermittent infusion dose, which is to be given centrally over 1 hour.

21 A 28-year-old man weighing 60 kg has taken an overdose of drug Y. Drug Y has a $t_{1/2}$ of 6 hours and the current serum level at 6 hours post-ingestion is 20 mg/L.
Calculate the amount of drug (mg/L) that will be eliminated from his body after 12 hours.

22 Calcium gluconate 10% injection (225 micromol/mL) is required for a patient undergoing hypocalcaemic tetany.
How many millimoles of calcium are contained in 10 mL of this preparation?

23 Calculate the weight (mg) of adrenaline contained in 20 mL of a 1 in 1000 solution.

24 Mrs W is a 93-year-old woman currently on regular morphine sulfate MR capsules at a dose of 60 mg BD. She also takes morphine sulfate 10 mg/5 mL oral solution at a dose of 10 mg every 4 hours PRN, which she has been taking on average four times a day. She is due to be switched to a subcutaneous syringe driver of diamorphine to help control her pain better.
What is the equivalent dose (mg) of diamorphine that Mrs W should be prescribed?

25 Zinc oxide spray is available as a 115-g aerosol and consists in part of the following ingredients: dimeticone 1.04% and zinc oxide 12.5% in a base containing wool alcohols, cetostearyl alcohol, dextran, white soft paraffin, liquid paraffin and propellants.
What is the weight (g) of zinc oxide (to one decimal place) in each bottle of this spray?

26 What weight (g) of potassium permanganate is required to produce 200 mL of a solution such that, when 50 mL of this solution is diluted to 500 mL, it will produce a 1 in 500 solution?

27 Child S, a 5-year-old girl with a BSA of $0.56\,m^2$, is being treated for eczema herpeticum using IV aciclovir. The recommended dose is $1.5\,g/m^2$ daily in three divided doses.
What dose (mg) of IV aciclovir should be prescribed for Child S?

28 Mr JW, a 37 year old weighing 72.45 kg, has just been started on IV human normal immunoglobulin at a dose of 0.4 g/kg per day for 5 days for the treatment of immune-mediated thrombocytopenia. The prescribing doctor decides to round the dose to the nearest 10-g dose.
Given that the product is available as 10-g vials, how many are needed to complete this treatment plan?

29 You are responding to an emergency cardiac arrest situation on the paediatric ward area. The doctor requests some sodium bicarbonate 4.2% for use to treat metabolic acidosis secondary to the cardiac arrest.

The nursing staff can only locate 8.4% due to a national shortage of the 4.2% product.
Given that the doctor requires 40 mL of a 4.2% sodium bicarbonate solution, what volume (mL) of the 8.4% solution must be mixed with water for injection to attain the desired concentration?

30 You are working on the manufacture of a new 400-mg antibiotic tablet formulation. During the manufacturing process you analyse the tolerance levels of the active ingredient and find it to be ±8%. What is the accepted maximum amount of active ingredient (mg) that a single tablet may contain?

# Best of five answers

## SECTION A

1 E

See BNF, Chapter 12, section 3.6. Mrs G probably has acute oral thrush precipitated by her newly prescribed *Symbicort*, which contains budesonide. Initial treatment should be with nystatin topically before using fluconazole systemically

2 A

*Symbicort* is a dry powder inhaler and should be inhaled quickly and deeply to ensure adequate delivery to the lungs. For more guidance on inhaler technique please see the relevant CPPE resources

3 C

See BNF, section 3.2. Oral thrush can be prevented by rinsing the mouth after using steroid-containing inhalers

4 A

Modified-release preparations should not be crushed as this can cause dose dumping. A select few modified-release formulations can be dispersed but specialist literature is needed to confirm this

5 E

See SPC, section 4.4. Clozapine can lead to agranulocytosis, neutropenia and depleted white blood cells. It is imperative that Mr F's white cell count is in range during therapy

6 C
See SPC, section 4.5. Alcohol can cause sedation, which may compound any sedation caused by clozapine. Patients should be warned about this and advised appropriately. Whilst it is ideal that patients with mental health conditions do not drink, this is not always achievable and the patient should be supported in making informed decisions and what could happen if they do drink

7 D
See SPC, section 4.2. Mr F has missed more than 48 hours of treatment and his clozapine will need to be re-initiated. A discussion with the specialist/prescriber is needed to determine the entire re-initiation programme

8 B
See BNF, Chapter 5, section 2. Oral metronidazole should be used first line in the first episode of *C. difficile* infection



9 C
See BNF, Chapter 5, section 2. See notes on superinfection

10 C
See BNF, Chapter 1, section 4.2. PPIs have been indicated as increasing the incidence of *C. difficile*

11 E
See BNF, Appendix 3, Cautionary and advisory labels for dispensed medicines and counselling information in the BNF monograph for doxycyline

12 D
See BNF, Chapter 2, section 8. Loop diuretics can be used twice daily, but to avoid disturbing sleep the second dose should be given no later than 4 pm

13 C
See MEP 38, section 3.3.10.2. As well as the usual label requirements, the words 'emergency supply' need to appear on the label

14 A
Using the BNF monograph for gabapentin, the maximum dose for a 10 year old is 300 mg (not 350 mg as per the 10 mg/kg dosing). 300 mg TDS on day 1 should be used for monotherapy only in children over 12 years of age

15 B
See BNF, Chapter 4, section 2.4. See the BNF monograph for mirtazapine and associated notices about blood disorders

16 C
See BNF, Chapter 7, section 1.2. Whilst option F is also correct, it is not always achievable in practice due to lack of suitable formulations

17 C
The image shows dry scaly skin with no obvious signs of infection (regardless, option B is a POM). This patient will probably benefit from a simple emollient such as *Diprobase*

18 C
See BNF, section 2.8.2, notes on management of high INR and minor bleeding. Note pharmacology of warfarin and management of high INR

19 A
See RPS guidance on the drugs and driving legislation

20 C
See palliative care guidance in the BNF. Lactulose (regularly) and senna (regularly/PRN) are commonly used in patients experiencing opioid- and immobility-induced (e.g. hospitalisation) constipation

21 D
See BNF, Chapter 1, section 8, Lipase Inhibitors, Orlistat, Multivitamins

22 D
See BNF, Chapter 2, section 4.1, risks of using beta blockers in diabetic patients

23 A
See NICE guidance on hypertension (CG127). Mr U's ethnicity means a calcium channel blocker should be used first line

24 A
See BNF, Chapter 2, section 1. Although rare, formation of ocular micro-deposits should be investigated by a specialist. Being dazzled by bright lights is a key sign of this

25 B
See BNF, Chapter 9, section 1.4. If caused by a bleed the stools would be described as tarry in consistency, so options A and E are ruled out

26 C
See SPC, section 4.2. Ciprofloxacin should be infused over 60 minutes

27 A
See SPC, section 6.2. Ciprofloxacin is not compatible with heparin. However, IV lines hold only small volumes so flushing the line with 10 mL of compatible solution will remove ciprofloxacin from the lumen, allowing it to be locked with the heparin solution

28 C
*Martindale: The Complete Drug Reference* will contain the international and street names of most drugs/medicines and should be the first resource you consult

29 C
See BNFC, section 4.6. Monograph for metoclopramide states that it is contraindicated in individuals who have had gastrointestinal surgery within the past 3–4 days. This is due to the pharmacology of metoclopramide

30 A
See BNFC, section 13.9. Cradle cap can be treated with olive or coconut oil, or a simple emollient. For more information on identifying cradle cap consult the book *Minor Illness or Major Disease*, 6th edn (Addison B *et al.*; Pharmaceutical Press, 2016)

## SECTION B

1 B

See BNF Chapter 6, section 4. Tablets should be swallowed whole. Doses should be taken with plenty of water while sitting or standing, on an empty stomach at least 30 minutes before breakfast (or another medicine); patient should stand or sit upright for at least 30 minutes after administration

2 E

See appropriate monographs and interactions in BNF for aspirin, dabigatran, lithium and methotrexate. All of them should not be used with NSAIDs. There are no issues with pizotifen

3 D

See *FASTtrack: Law and Ethics in Pharmacy Practice*

4 D

See BNF, Chapter 2, section 3.2 for more about warfarin; for tablet colours refer to SPC or product packaging. The colours are 1 mg brown, 3 mg blue and 5 mg pink. The colours of warfarin tablets are the same across the world. Always ask patients what colour and strength they are expecting when dispensing

5 C

See any first-aid book. Always cool the burn first and then dress it. Blisters should never be popped and creams, ointments and fats should not be applied. The burn is not big or serious enough to warrant an ambulance

6 D

See BNF, Appendix 1 (Interactions) under Trimethoprim

7 A

See BNF, Chapter 7, section 4.2. *Priligy* (dapoxetine) is the only drug available for this indication currently

8 A

See BNF, Chapter 12, section 1.1. Alclometasone is not available as an ear preparation; it is available as a cream

**9 B**
See BNF, Chapter 12, section 1.1. Clioquinol stains skin and clothing

**10 A**
See BNF, Chapter 12, section 1.2, under Removal of ear wax. *Cerumol* contains arachis (peanut) oil

**11 E**
See BNF, Chapter 13, section 1. *Hydromol* does not contain urea

**12 A**
See BNF, Chapter 13, section 3. *Modrasone* is the same potency as *Eumovate*

**13 C**
See BNF, Chapter 7, section 1.1. Mirabegron is a beta-3-adrenoceptor agonist (i.e. not an antimuscarinic drug). It is recommended by NICE as an option only for patients in whom antimuscarinic drugs are ineffective, contraindicated or not tolerated

**14 E**
See BNF, Appendix 1, Interactions and Daktarin Oral Gel SPC

**15 E**
See *Chemist & Druggist Guide to OTC Medicines and Diagnostics*. HC45 1% cream and *Eumovate* eczema/dermatitis cream are 1% hydrocortisone and 0.05% clobetasone butryrate, respectively. Hydrocortisone 1% cream is also available generically

**16 B**
See *FASTtrack: Managing Symptoms in the Pharmacy*. They should be used only in patients over 18 years of age

**17 A**
See *FASTtrack: Managing Symptoms in the Pharmacy*. Bismuth oxide is an astringent. Cinchocaine is a local anaesthetic. Mucopolysaccharide polysulfate is a fibrinolytic agent. Shark liver oil is a skin protectant. Yeast cell extract is a wound-healing agent

18 D
See *FASTtrack: Managing Symptoms in the Pharmacy*. Potassium bicarbonate can cause hyperkalaemia

19 D
See *FASTtrack: Managing Symptoms in the Pharmacy*. It should be left on for 8–12 hours. If hands are washed during that time, then the cream should be applied again

20 C
See *FASTtrack: Managing Symptoms in the Pharmacy*. *Lamisil Once* contains terbinafine. Both feet should be treated even if lesions are visible on one foot only. For best results, the treated area should not be washed for 24 hours after application

21 B
See BNF Chapter 2, section 6. Colestid may delay or reduce the absorption of certain concomitant drugs

22 D
See *Chemist & Druggist Guide to OTC Medicines and Diagnostics*. There is little evidence to show that rice-based formulas are more effective than glucose-based oral rehydration therapy

23 C
See *FASTtrack: Managing Symptoms in the Pharmacy*. *Dioralyte* can be recommended as well as referral to GP. The child is at risk of dehydration

24 E
See MEP guide or RPS quick reference guide titled 'European Economic Area (EEA) prescriptions'

25 E
See *FASTtrack: Managing Symptoms in the Pharmacy*. Abdominal pain, bloating, constipation and diarrhoea are common in IBS. Vomiting is not

26 A
See *FASTtrack: Managing Symptoms in the Pharmacy*. Acetic acid is available in a preparation for ears

27 E
See *FASTtrack: Managing Symptoms in the Pharmacy*. Naproxen is licensed OTC from 15 years of age

28 B
See MEP guide. Isotretinoin prescriptions are valid only for 7 days

29 E
See *FASTtrack: Managing Symptoms in the Pharmacy*. Hyoscine lasts for 4 hours, promethazine hydrochloride 6–8 hours and cinnarizine 8 hours

30 D
See *FASTtrack: Managing Symptoms in the Pharmacy*. Hyoscine causes the least sedation. Promethazine teoclate and cinnarizine cause a similar amount of sedation

31 D
See *FASTtrack: Managing Symptoms in the Pharmacy*. See explanation for question 29

32 D
See SPC, section 5.2, Pharmacokinetic properties. Following cessation of dosing, approximately 95% of topically applied minoxidil will be eliminated within 4 days

33 A
See SPC, section 4.2, Posology and method of administration. The total dosage should not exceed 2 mL

34 C
See SPC, section 4.9, Overdose. 100 mg is the maximum recommended adult dose for oral minoxidil administration in the treatment of hypertension

35 E
See SPC, section 4.4, Special warnings and precautions for use. It should be used with caution in narrow-angle glaucoma

36 A
See SPC, section 5.2, Pharmacokinetic properties. Only about 1% of a single dose is excreted unchanged in urine

37 D

See SPC, section 5.2, Pharmacokinetic properties. The sedative effect appears to be maximal within 1–3 hours after administration of a single dose

38 A

See SPCs for each product. *Daktarin Sugar Free Oral Gel* is licensed from 3 months. *Piriton* syrup is licensed from 12 months. *Germoloids* HC spray is licensed from 16 years. *Beconase Hayfever Relief* nasal spray is licensed from 18 years. *Regaine for Men Extra Strength* is licensed only up until 65 years

39 B

See *Nexium Control* SPC. *Nexium Control* is esomeprazole. The OTC dose is 20 mg once daily. It is licensed for the short-term treatment of reflux symptoms in adults

40 B

The symptoms describe chickenpox. There are no reasons to refer in this scenario. The rash appears to be getting worse in the eyes of the parent but this is just the progression of symptoms of chickenpox. An appropriate OTC product should be recommended to help with the symptoms, e.g. calamine lotion and/or chlorphenamine solution. You could refer to the GP but that would not be the most appropriate option as it can be dealt with in the pharmacy. See *Minor Illness or Major Disease*, 6th edn (Addison B *et al.*; Pharmaceutical Press, 2016)

## SECTION C

1 B
See BNF, section 4, Nausea and labyrinth disorders under Motion sickness. Antiemetics should be given to prevent motion sickness rather than after nausea or vomiting develop. The most effective drug for the prevention of motion sickness is hyoscine hydrobromide

2 E
Mr L is suffering from otitis externa, also known as swimmer's ear. The characteristic symptom is itching. Other common symptoms include pain, inflammation and tenderness of the ear. Conductive hearing loss is not a referral point as it can also occur if there is severe swelling of the ear canal. Profuse mucopurulent discharge is associated with otitis media

3 D
See MHRA website: https://www.gov.uk/advertise-your-medicines#adverts-for-medicines-definition

4 B
Not all material that is published in a journal is considered a primary resource. Original clinical trials are considered primary literature; however, periodicals, review articles, articles of opinion, correspondence and special reports are not. http://research.library.gsu.edu/c.php?g=115556&p=752623

5 E
The supply of health promotional material surrounding disease states is considered educational material. See MHRA website: https://www.gov.uk/advertise-your-medicines#adverts-for-medicines-definition

6 D
See BNF, section 14.4

7 C
Symptoms are consistent with plaque psoriasis, which is the most common form. Only plaque and scalp psoriasis can be treated in a community pharmacy. See *Community Pharmacy*, 3rd edn (Rutter P; Churchill Livingstone, 2013)

8 C

Highly osmotic solutions of glucose, such as soda, may result in more water being absorbed into the intestinal tract and exacerbating diarrhoea. In many cases, diarrhoea will resolve within 48 hours without treatment; however, in severe cases of infectious diarrhoea it may be treated with antibiotics

9 D

Due to the beta-adrenergic-blocking effects of metoprolol (e.g. decreased heart rate, decreased blood pressure, decreased inotropic effect), there is a net decrease in myocardial oxygen demand. The opposite effect is seen in isoprenaline, which is a beta agonist. Cold temperatures increase the myocardial oxygen demand by increasing sympathetic stimulation, systolic blood pressure and cardiac diastolic pressure, and volume

10 A

See BNF, Chapter 1, section 1.2. Bisacodyl acts within 10–12 hours, docusate sodium acts within 24–48 hours and lactulose may take up to 48 hours. Ispaghula husk 'full effect may take days to develop'. Note: senna acts within 8–12 hours

11 C

See BNF, Chapter 4, section 5.1. Sumatriptan should not be administered to patients with severe hepatic impairment. Liver disease does not indicate severe impairment. Sumatriptan is contraindicated in patients who have ischaemic heart disease or have had a myocardial infarction, coronary vasospasm (Prinzmetal's angina), peripheral vascular disease, or symptoms or signs consistent with ischaemic heart disease. It should also not be administered to patients with a history of cerebrovascular accident (CVA) or transient ischaemic attack (TIA), or to patients with moderate and severe hypertension and mild uncontrolled hypertension. Sumatriptan causes vasoconstriction; this effect when present in coronary vessels may cause chest tightness as a normal side-effect. However, in patients with ischaemic heart disease, angina or a risk of coronary artery disease, this could precipitate attacks of angina or potentially cause myocardial infarction, and thus should not be used in these patients

12 E
See BNF, Guidance on prescribing, Adverse Reactions to Drugs, Teeth and Jaw. Intrinsic staining of teeth is most commonly caused by tetracyclines. Effects on teeth may be seen if given at any time from about the fourth month *in utero* until the age of 12 years. All tetracyclines may cause permanent unsightly staining in children, varying from yellow to grey. Chlorhexidine may stain teeth brown but can easily be removed by polishing. Iron salts in liquid form can stain the enamel black. Superficial staining has been reported rarely with co-amoxiclav suspension. Excessive ingestion of fluoride leads to dental fluorosis with mottling (white patches) of the enamel and areas of hypoplasia or pitting

13 D
See BNF, Guidance on prescribing, Adverse Reactions to Drugs, Oral side-effects of drugs. The oral mucosa is particularly vulnerable to ulceration in patients treated with cytotoxic drugs, e.g. methotrexate. Other drugs that are capable of causing oral ulceration include ACE inhibitors, gold, nicorandil, NSAIDs, pancreatin, pencillamine, proguanil and protease inhibitors. Aspirin tablets allowed to dissolve in the sulcus for the treatment of toothache can lead to a white patch followed by ulceration. Propranolol is a beta blocker that has not been shown to cause aphthous ulcers

14 D
Spironolactone is a weak diuretic that has shown to be beneficial to patients with moderate-to-severe symptoms of heart failure by its direct antagonistic effect on aldosterone

15 C
See MEP guide and PSNC website: http://psnc.org.uk/services-commissioning/advanced-services/

16 D
See BNF, Emergency treatment of poisoning. Renal tubular necrosis may occur but much less frequently

**17 E**

Oral anticoagulants act by inhibiting the liver biosynthesis of prothrombin, which is the precursor of the enzyme thrombin that catalyses the conversion of soluble fibrinogen to the insoluble polymer fibrin, resulting in clot formation. One of the principal factors in the biosynthesis of prothrombin is vitamin K, with which warfarin competes to inhibit this process. Vitamin K thus acts as an antagonist to the oral anticoagulants through reversible competition

**18 B**

See BNF, Emergency treatment of poisoning, Calcium-channel blockers. Parenteral calcium is used to reverse the cardiac effects of calcium-channel blocker overdose and hyperkalaemia

**19 A**

See BNF, section 8.1.4. Vinblastine, vincristine, vindesine, vinflunine and vinorelbine injections are for intravenous administration only. Inadvertent intrathecal administration can cause severe neurotoxicity, which is usually fatal

**20 C**

See BNF, Chapter 3, section 4, MHRA/CHM Advice (March 2008/2009). Demulcent cough preparations contain soothing substances, such as syrup or glycerol, and some patients believe that such preparations relieve a dry irritating cough. Preparations such as simple linctus have the advantage of being harmless and inexpensive; paediatric simple linctus is particularly useful in children. Compound preparations are on sale to the public for the treatment of coughs and colds but should not be used in children under 6 years; the rationale for some is dubious. Care should be taken to give the correct dose and not to use more than one preparation at a time; see MHRA/CHM advice

**21 C**

Evaluation is a step in the CPD cycle. See http://www.smoking2.nes.scot.nhs.uk/module2/cycle-of-change.html

**22 D**

Hydrocortisone can be used only in adults and children over 10 years of age. Chlorphenamine (>1 year), crotamiton (>3 years), lidocaine (>4 years), ammonia 3.5% w/w (>2 years). See *Community Pharmacy*, 3rd edn (Rutter P; Churchill Livingstone, 2013)

23 A

Vulvovaginal sores are indicative of herpes infection. See http://www.nhs.uk/Conditions/Chlamydia/Pages/Symptoms.aspx

24 E

Tamsulosin is used for benign prostatic hyperplasia (BPH) in which the prostate gland is enlarged and responsible for urinary symptoms. Uncontrolled or undiagnosed diabetes can cause damage to the autonomic nervous system which, among other things, controls bladder function. This damage can lead to urinary frequency (which is also a symptom of BPH), but other symptoms that may be present with uncontrolled or undiagnosed diabetes include excessive thirst and tiredness. Tamsulosin should not be given to men who experience postural hypotension because, as with other alpha-1 blockers, a reduction in blood pressure can occur in some people during treatment with tamsulosin

25 C

See BNF Chapter 2, section 2, Antifibrinolytic drugs and haemostatics. Tranexamic acid is indicated for the reduction of heavy menstrual bleeding over several cycles in women with regular 21- to 35-day cycles with no more than 3 days' individual variability in cycle duration for women of 18 years and above. Patient criteria for OTC sale differ from use with prescription. Note that tranexamic acid when prescribed may be used with caution in patients with irregular menstrual bleeding according to the BNF. However, patients with more than 3 days of menstrual cycle variability are not eligible for OTC sale of tranexamic acid

26 A

Rewetting solutions are the only contact lens solutions that may be used while the lens is still in the eye. See *Clinical Contact Lens Practice* (Bennett ES, Weissman BA, eds; Lippincott Williams & Wilkins, 2005)

27 A

Octyl methoxycinnamate and homosalate protect only against UVB exposure. Photosensitivity reactions most often result from UVA radiation exposure. See http://www.skincancer.org/prevention/sun-protection/sunscreen/the-skin-cancer-foundations-guide-to-sunscreens

28 E
See BNF, Chapter 6, section 3.1. Should be continued only if HbA1c concentration is reduced by at least 0.5 percentage points within 6 months of starting treatment

29 C
See *Community Pharmacy*, 3rd edn (Rutter P; Churchill Livingstone, 2013)

30 A
See BNF, Emergency Treatment of Poisoning, Specific drugs, Analgesics (non-opioid)

31 E
Checking manufacturer's name is not part of the dispensing process and is least likely to reduce dispensing errors comparatively

32 E
See BNF, Chapter 8, section 2.6, Tamoxifen. Tamoxifen may increase the risk of endometrial cancer. It increases the efficacy of warfarin and therefore increases susceptibility to high INR readings. Timing of tamoxifen will not reduce the hot flush which is a common side-effect. Tamoxifen increases the risk of venous thromboembolism and a swollen leg could suggest a deep vein thrombosis, which requires urgent medical attention in a hospital

33 B
There is no conclusive evidence that prolonged exposure to sunlight or using sunbeds or sunlamps can improve acne. Many medications used to treat acne may sensitise skin to light; thus exposure could cause painful damage

34 B
The patient has allergic rhinitis, which is differentiated from the common cold by the nasal itching. Pseudoephedrine and *Breathe Right Nasal Strips* are indicated for nasal congestion, which she does not have. Both chlorphenamine and intranasal sodium cromoglicate are recommended for relief of sneezing and rhinorrhoea in pregnancy. However, with sodium cromoglicate it will take 1–2 weeks for symptoms to improve whilst chlorphenamine will provide relief within hours. Therefore, chlorphenamine

is the best choice for this patient. Most manufacturers of antihistamines advise avoiding their use during pregnancy; however, there is no evidence of teratogenicity except for hydroxyzine for which toxicity has been reported with high doses in animal studies. The use of sedating antihistamines in the latter part of the third trimester may cause adverse effects in neonates, such as irritability, paradoxical excitability and tremor. See *Community Pharmacy* 3rd edn (Rutter P; Churchill Livingstone, 2013)

35 E
See BNF, Chapter 7, section 1.2 under Patient and carer advice. Also see Appendix 3 Cautionary and advisory labels

36 D
See BNF, Chapter 13, section 8.1. Minoxidil 5% scalp solution (*Regaine*) is used to treat androgenetic alopecia (balding) and is not available on an NHS prescription

37 E
See BNF, Chapter 1, section 4.1 under Simeticone. Symptoms are consistent with colic

38 C
See BNF, Chapter 5, section 2.6 under Urinary-tract infections – Nitrofurantoin monograph under cautions states 'urine may be coloured yellow or brown'

39 E
See BNF, section 5.1.6. Patients should discontinue immediately and contact doctor if diarrhoea develops because clindamycin has been associated with antibiotic-associated colitis (see BNF, section 1.5), which may be fatal. It is most common in middle-aged and elderly women, especially following an operation. Although antibiotic-associated colitis can occur with most antibacterials, it occurs more frequently with clindamycin

40 A
Prophylactic enoxaparin is contraindicated following an acute stroke (for at least 2 months but varies according to hospital)

41 E
See SPC, section 4.4, Special warnings and precautions for use under 'Surgery'. As *Janumet* contains metformin hydrochloride, the treatment should be discontinued 48 hours before elective surgery with general, spinal or epidural anaesthesia. Treatment should not usually be resumed earlier than 48 hours afterwards and only after renal function has been re-evaluated and found to be normal

42 B
See SPC, section 4.4, Special warnings and precautions for use under 'Administration of iodinated contrast agent'. The intravascular administration of iodinated contrast agents in radiological studies can lead to renal failure, which has been associated with lactic acidosis in patients receiving metformin. Therefore, treatment should be discontinued prior to, or at the time of, the test and not reinstituted until 48 hours afterwards, and only after renal function has been re-evaluated and found to be normal (see section 4.5)

43 E
See SPC, section 4.3. Not contraindicated in mild renal impairment, only in moderate and severe renal impairment (creatinine clearance <60 mL/minute) (see section 4.4)

44 B
See SPC, section 4.8 under 'Undesirable effects'

45 C
See SPC, section 4.5, Interaction with other medicinal products and other forms of interaction. St John's wort increases the effects of tolbutamide, which may lead to increased hypoglycaemic events, whereas extracts of ginkgo biloba may decrease absorption of tolbutamide and thereby decrease its efficacy and hypoglycaemic effect

46 C
See SPC, section 4.5, Interaction with other medicinal products and other forms of interaction. Alcohol may increase hypoglycaemic effects and may also cause a disulfiram-like reaction. See also section 4.8, Undesirable effects. Paraesthesiae and headaches have been reported. Patients may become intolerant to alcohol and should limit intake

## SECTION D

1 C
Refer to a good OTC or responding to symptoms textbook

2 C
Child is allergic to penicillin, hence a macrolide is the drug of choice

3 C
See BNFC, Chapter 13, section 2 and Chapter 5, section 2 (Bacterial Infection – summary tables)

4 E
See Drug Tariff extract for more detail

5 C
See responsible pharmacist legislation and note the difference in duties between a responsible pharmacist and a superintendent pharmacist

6 D
See MHRA guidance on reporting of dispensing errors. Note: it is not a must to review the SOP unless it was a factor in the error occurring

7 D
Refer to a good therapeutics textbook

8 C
See BNFC, Chapter 1, section 10 for more information

9 D
See MEP guide

10 A
Liposomal amphotericin is compatible only in glucose 5% (see SPC for more detail)

11 C
See SPC for more detail

12 B
See SPC for more detail and also apply your pharmacy and therapeutics knowledge to the situation

13 B
See BNF, Chapter 6, section 3.1. Risk of lactic acidosis if metformin not withheld

14 D
See BNF, Appendix 1, Interactions under statins. Increased plasma concentration of atorvastatin when used alongside clarithromycin can lead to myopathy

15 D
See BNF, Chapter 6, section 4. Bone and mineral electrolytes need to be checked (e.g. calcium, vitamin D and phosphate)

16 C
See BNF, Chapter 6, section 4. Dental examination needed due to risk of osteonecrosis

17 D
See BNF, Chapter 6, section 4. Heartburn can be a sign of oesophageal reactions

18 B
See BNF extract provided. The range of acceptable infusion concentration is 0.5–2.5 mg/mL

19 C
Codeine is contraindicated in patients following adeno-tonsillectomy procedures. See associated MHRA/CHM advice in BNFC, Chapter 4, section 4

20 E
Codeine can cause respiratory depression and problems in those who are unable to metabolise it. See associated MHRA/CHM advice in BNFC, Chapter 4, section 4

21 C
A positive D-dimer result indicates a treatment dose of a low-molecular-weight heparin product is needed

22 B
A high INR indicates that the blood is not clotting as quickly as it should be

23 A
See BNF, Chapter 2, section 3.2, under Vitamin K antagonists for more information relating to dietary effects. Diet should not be changed drastically as it will affect the anticoagulation effect of warfarin

24 D
See MEP guide, section 3.3.1, General prescription requirements

25 D
See BNF, Chapter 2, section 4.1. ACEIs can cause a persistent dry cough

26 A
See BNF, Chapter 2, section 8. In resistant oedema, the dose of furosemide should be increased to maximum for this indication, which is 120 mg daily

27 D
Prednisolone, salbutamol and furosemide can all lower potassium levels

28 A
Refer to NICE Clinical Guidance 92 (CG92) on VTE prophylaxis

29 E
A family history of cardiac disease does not necessarily increase risk of VTE; however, if a patient has a cardiac co-morbidity, this would increase risk

30 E
Refer to diagram and own knowledge; mechanical prophylaxis refers to stockings, hosiery, etc.

# *Extended matching answers*

**SECTION A**

1 E
See interaction between simvastatin and erythromycin. Concurrent use is contraindicated so the patient should withhold simvastatin while on erythromycin

2 D
See BNFC, section 5.1.3. Tetracyclines should be avoided in children under 12 years of age owing to their ability to interfere with bone development

3 C
See interaction between spironolactone and trimethoprim (which is in co-trimoxazole); risk of hyperkalaemia when given together

4 G
See interaction between metronidazole and alcohol. This is of more clinical relevance than for the other drugs listed, even though the effect on alcohol for these is also worth knowing

5 A
See BNF, Chapter 5, section 2, under Quinolones

6 H
See BNF, Chapter 4, section 2.4; notes on withdrawal and which drugs are most associated with withdrawal symptoms and why

7 B
See BNF, Chapter 4, section 2.4; notes under choice and management, which indicate SSRIs as first-line agents

8 F
See BNF, Chapter 4, section 2.4; notes on interactions between antidepressants and further notes in the SSRI and reversible MAOI sections

9 F
See BNF, Chapter 4, section 2.4; notes on interaction between MAOIs and certain foods, a number of which may be common in Asian diets

10 H
See BNF, Chapter 8, section 2.2; important note regarding the administration of vinca alkaloids

11 F
See BNF, Chapter 8, section 2.2; notes on urothelial toxicity. Oncology is a complex specialism but you may be expected to know key details about these medicines and identify cytotoxic agents from non-cytotoxic agents



12 B
See BNF, Chapter 2, section 6; counselling notes for acid sequestrants

13 D
See BNF, Chapter 2, section 6. Blood triglyceride concentration should be less than 1.8 mmol/L. A fibrate can be added to a statin to reduce triglycerides when a statin fails to do so

14 A
See BNF, Chapter 2, section 6. Statins are the first-line option for reducing cardiac risk in patients with high cholesterol. Note the interaction between amiodarone and simvastatin in the BNF (patients should still be monitored for myopathy if atorvastatin has been started; see *Stockley's Drug Interactions*, 11th edn (Preston CL, ed; Pharmaceutical Press, 2016) for more information) and NICE Clinical Guideline 181 (favours atorvastatin)

15 B
See BNF, Chapter 2, section 6; notes on hypercholesterolaemia and also the introductory notes for the ezetimibe monograph

16 A
See BNF, Chapter 9, section 6. Vitamin D aids the absorption of calcium. Note this patient has renal disease so will need the activated form of vitamin $D_3$

17 E
See BNF, Chapter 9, section 1.5. A total gastrectomy is complete removal of the stomach and these patients need supplementation with vitamin $B_{12}$

18 H
See BNF, Chapter 9, section 6; risks in pregnancy

19 G
See BNF, Chapter 9, section 6. *Pabrinex* is a vitamin B complex that is used in the initial management of Wernicke's encephalopathy. This should be changed to oral thiamine when clinically appropriate

20 C
See BNF, Chapter 14, section 4. Candidates should know that *Fluenz Tetra* is the live attenuated flu vaccine, which is given intranasally and is referred to in the excerpt provided with the question. This vaccine is contraindicated in those who will come into close contact with immunocompromised patients, so the injection (*Fluarix Tetra*) would be most appropriate

21 F
See BNF, section 14.4; notes on use of tetanus immunoglobulins after injury

22 I
Mr G is exhibiting warning signs (unexplained weight loss) and should be referred to his GP. See Chapter 8 of *Minor Illness or Major Disease*, 6th edn (Addison B *et al.*; Pharmaceutical Press, 2016)

23 A
The child is responsive and no other warning signs are described. Whilst the number of stools is not too worrying, his dry lips would make oral rehydration the most plausible option. See sections 1.4 and 9.2.1.2 of the BNFC and also Chapter 2 of *Minor Illness or Major Disease*, 6th edn (Addison B *et al.*; Pharmaceutical Press, 2016)

ANSWERS

**24 F**
The spicy food may have triggered the dyspepsia and heartburn, and therefore an alginate product would be an appropriate first choice. Consider referring the patient if the alginate product does not work. See Chapter 2 of *Minor Illness or Major Disease*, 6th edn (Addison B *et al.*; Pharmaceutical Press, 2016)

**25 H**
Constipation is fairly common and warrants treatment only in patients who feel the effects of constipation, or have been constipated for longer (7–14 days). See Chapter 2 of *Minor Illness or Major Disease*, 6th edn (Addison B *et al.*; Pharmaceutical Press, 2016)

**26 G**
Mrs K should try senna as this is much faster acting than lactulose. If her constipation does not resolve within 4 days, or she develops stomach pains, she should see her GP. See Chapter 2 of *Minor Illness or Major Disease*, 6th edn (Addison B *et al.*; Pharmaceutical Press, 2016)

**27 F**
See BNF, Chapter 1, section 4.3. Gastro-oesophageal reflux is common in the later stages of pregnancy as the fetus gets larger. These symptoms can respond well to alginate products, which can be taken throughout the day and also at night

**28 E**
See BNF, Chapter 6, section 4. Alendronate should be taken this way to prevent oesophagitis

**29 D**
See BNF, Appendix 3. Lansoprazole should be taken 30–60 minutes before food

**30 F**
See BNF, Appendix 3. Flucloxacillin should be taken on an empty stomach

## SECTION B

1 F
See Drug Safety Update (July 2015)

2 H
See BNF, Chapter 11, section 5. Beta blockers should be avoided in uncontrolled heart failure

3 F
See BNF, Chapter 11, section 5. Latanoprost can cause eyelashes to become darker, thicker and longer

4 A
See BNF, Chapter 11, section 5

5 G
See BNF, Chapter 11, section 5. Blurred vision due to pilocarpine may affect performance of skilled tasks (e.g. driving), particularly at night or in reduced lighting

6 D
See BNF, Chapter 3, section 1. Indacaterol is a long-acting beta agonist (LABA) and is available as *Onbrez Breezhaler*

7 E
See BNF, Chapter 3, section 1. Olodaterol is a LABA and is available as *Striverdi Respimat*

8 A
See BNF, Chapter 3, section 1. Aclidinium is a long-acting muscarinic antagonist (LAMA) and is available as *Eklira Genuair*

9 C
See BNF, Chapter 3, section 1. Glycopyrronium is a LAMA and is available as *Seebri Breezhaler*

10 H
See BNF, Chapter 3, section 1. Umeclidinium is a LAMA and is available as *Incruse Ellipta*

11 B
See BNF, Chapter 7, section 3.4. *Depo-Provera* is repeated every 12 weeks

12 C
See BNF, Chapter 7, section 3.3. *ellaOne* is licensed for up to 120 hours after coitus

13 A
See BNF, Chapter 7, section 3.3. Desogestrel has a 12-hour window before contraceptive cover may be lost. Other drugs in the same class have a 3-hour window

14 G
See BNF, Chapter 7, section 3.1. *Qlaira* is an everyday phasic preparation

15 H
See BNF, Chapter 7, section 3.1. *Zoely* is an everyday monophasic preparation

16 E
See BNF, Chapter 1, section 1. Linaclotide is a guanylate cyclase-C-receptor agonist that is licensed for the treatment of moderate-to-severe IBS associated with constipation

17 B
See BNF, Chapter 1, section 1. Dantron is indicated only for constipation in terminally ill patients of all ages. This is because of its potential carcinogenicity and evidence of genotoxicity

18 F
See BNF, Chapter 1, section 1. Liquid paraffin can cause anal seepage and consequent anal irritation after prolonged use

**19 D**
See BNF, Chapter 1, section 1. Lactulose produces an osmotic diarrhoea of low faecal pH and discourages the proliferation of ammonia-producing organisms. It is therefore useful in the treatment of hepatic encephalopathy

**20 C**
See BNF, Chapter 1, section 1. If dietary and lifestyle changes fail to control constipation in pregnancy, moderate doses of poorly absorbed laxatives may be used. A bulk-forming laxative should be tried first

**21 F**
See BNF, Chapter 6, section 3. Nateglinide has a maximum dose of 180 mg TDS. It stimulates insulin secretion

**22 B**
See BNF, Chapter 6, section 3. Vildagliptin is licensed in over-18s as triple therapy with metformin and sulfonylureas

**23 G**
See BNF, Chapter 6, section 3. Tolbutamide is a short-acting sulfonylurea. Long-acting sulfonylureas should be avoided in the elderly

**24 H**
See BNF, Chapter 6, section 3. Insulin degludec is available as 100 units/mL and 200 units/mL. Ensure correct strength is prescribed and dispensed

**25 C**
See BNF, Chapter 6, section 3. Canagliflozin reversibly inhibits sodium–glucose co-transporter 2 in the renal proximal convoluted tubule, to reduce glucose reabsorption and increase urinary glucose excretion. As such, UTIs may occur

**26 C**
See BNF, Chapter 4, section 8. Bupropion should be discontinued if abstinence is not achieved after 7 weeks

**27 D**

See BNF, Chapter 4, section 8. Disulfiram gives rise to an extremely unpleasant systemic reaction after the ingestion of even a small amount of acetaldehyde into the body

**28 G**

See BNF, Chapter 4, section 8. See also NICE Technology appraisal guideline [TA325] November 2014

**29 E**

See BNF, Chapter 4, section 8. Lofexidine is licensed for the management of symptoms of opioid withdrawal

**30 H**

See BNF, Chapter 4, section 8. MHRA/CHM advice is to discontinue varenicline and seek prompt medical advice if patients develop agitation, depressed mood or suicidal thoughts

**31 H**

See BNF, Chapter 4, section 8.2. Patients can use one spray in each nostril when the urge to smoke occurs, up to twice every hour for 16 hours. Maximum 64 sprays daily, 32 in each nostril

**32 F**

See BNF, Chapter 4, section 8.2. Chew the gum until the taste becomes strong, then rest it between the cheek and gum; when the taste starts to fade, repeat this process. One piece of gum lasts for approximately 30 minutes

**33 G**

See BNF, Chapter 4, section 8.2. The amount of nicotine from one puff of the cartridge is less than that from a cigarette, and therefore it is necessary to inhale more often than when smoking a cigarette. A single 15-mg cartridge lasts for approximately 40 minutes of intense use

**34 G**
See BNF, Chapter 4, section 8.2. Individuals who smoke fewer than 20 cigarettes a day should initially use one tablet per hour, increased to two tablets each hour if necessary. Individuals who smoke more than 20 cigarettes each day should use two tablets each hour. Patients should not exceed 40 tablets daily

**35 E**
See BNF, Chapter 4, section 8.2. Patients should not exceed 12 cartridges of the 10 mg strength daily. A single 10-mg cartridge lasts for approximately 20 minutes of intense use

**36 E**
See Counter Intelligence Plus book (2016) or app (Apple or Android). Women aged 15–50 years: two (500 mg) tablets. If necessary another tablet can be taken 6–8 hours later. Maximum three (750 mg) tablets in 24 hours

**37 H**
See Counter Intelligence Plus book (2016) or app (Apple or Android). Over 16 years: two (525 mg) tablets every 30–60 minutes if needed, up to a maximum of 16 (4200 mg) in 24 hours

**38 C**
See Counter Intelligence Plus book (2016) or app (Apple or Android). Over 16 years and the elderly: one (75 mg) tablet as needed. If symptoms persist for more than 1 hour or return, another tablet can be taken. Maximum two (150 mg) tablets in 24 hours

**39 F**
See Counter Intelligence Plus book (2016) or app (Apple or Android). Either 6 × 200 mg or 3 × 400 mg (1200 mg) ibuprofen can be taken OTC daily

**40 B**
See Counter Intelligence Plus book (2016) or app (Apple or Android). Over 12 years: one lozenge every 3–6 hours as required. Max. five (43.75 mg) lozenges in 24 hours

ANSWERS

## SECTION C

1 H
See BNF, Chapter 11, section 4. Short-acting, relatively weak mydriatics, such as tropicamide 0.5% (action lasts for 4–6 hours), facilitate the examination of the fundus of the eye

2 G
See BNF, Chapter 11, section 5. Topical application of a beta blocker to the eye reduces intra-ocular pressure effectively in *primary open-angle glaucoma*, probably by reducing the rate of production of aqueous humour. Systemic absorption can follow topical application to the eyes; therefore, eye drops containing a beta blocker are contraindicated in patients with bradycardia, heart block or uncontrolled heart failure

3 B
Mucopurulent discharge is a classic symptom of bacterial conjunctivitis. Treat with chloramphenicol eye drops for a maximum of 5 days

4 E
Herpes simplex infections producing dendritic corneal ulcers can be treated with aciclovir or ganciclovir

5 F
Sodium cromoglicate is a prophylactic agent for the treatment of allergies and is safe for use in pregnant women

6 C
Classic symptoms of glandular fever include swollen glands, fever, malaise and headache, as well as a maculopapular rash which appears on the trunk

7 E
Measles – Koplik's spots and a rash first appear on ear and face and then progress to trunk and limbs. See *Community Pharmacy*, 3rd edn (Rutter P; Churchill Livingstone, 2013)

8 F
Meningitis – symptoms include fever, lethargy, stiff neck, vomiting, photophobia and a rash with purplish blotches. See *Community Pharmacy*, 3rd edn, p. 303 (Rutter P; Churchill Livingstone, 2013)

9 D
Impetigo – characteristic symptoms include vesicles that exude, forming yellow crusts around facial area, particularly nose and mouth. It is most common among school-aged children. See *Community Pharmacy*, 3rd edn, p. 303 (Rutter P; Churchill Livingstone, 2013)

10 D
See BNF, Chapter 13, section 2. In the community, acute impetigo on small areas of the skin may be treated by short-term topical application of fusidic acid. Impetigo is often caused by either *Staphylococcus aureus* or *Streptococcus pyogenes* through broken skin. Impetigo infection may occur through a breach in the skin and stops being infectious after 48 hours of treatment starting or after the sores have stopped blistering or crusting

11 H
See BNF, Chapter 1, section 2.2. Prucalopride is a selective serotonin $5HT_4$-receptor agonist with prokinetic properties

12 B
See BNF, Chapter 2, section 6, under Other drugs used in constipation. Colestyramine is an anion-exchange resin that is not absorbed from the gastrointestinal tract. It relieves diarrhoea and pruritus by forming an insoluble complex with bile acids in the intestine

13 D
Lactulose may be used to treat constipation in children. See *Community Pharmacy*, 3rd edn (Rutter P; Churchill Livingstone, 2013)

14 F
See BNF, Chapter 1, section 2.1, under Drugs affecting biliary composition and flow. Bowel cleansing preparations, e.g. *MoviPrep* and *KleanPrep*, are prescribed for bowel evacuation before colonoscopy or surgery

**15 A**
See BNF, Chapter 1, section 2.2. Bisacodyl tablets act in 10–12 hours

**16 G**
See BNF, Chapter 1, section 4.2. Omeprazole is used in conjunction with amoxicillin 500 mg three times daily and metronidazole 400 mg three times daily as triple therapy for *Helicobacter pylori* eradication

**17 B**
See BNF, Chapter 1, section 7.1 and Medical Emergencies in the Community. Aspirin (chewed or dispersed in water) is given for its antiplatelet effect (BNF section 2.9); a dose of 300 mg is suitable. If aspirin is given before arrival at hospital, a note saying that it has been given should be sent with the patient

**18 A**
See BNF, Chapter 2, section 1 under Antiarrhythmics. Amiodarone is used in the treatment of arrhythmias, particularly when other drugs are ineffective or contraindicated

**19 E**
See BNF, Chapter 8, section 2.2 under Monitoring requirements

**20 G**
See BNF, Chapter 3, section 1 under Monitoring requirements. Adverse effects can occur within the range 10–20 mg/L and both the frequency and severity increase at concentrations above 20 mg/L

**21 C**
See BNF, Chapter 2, section 1 under Dose equivalence and conversion. When switching from intravenous to oral route, dose may need to be increased by 20–33% to maintain the same plasma-digoxin concentration. Digoxin doses in the BNF may differ from those in product literature. For plasma concentration monitoring, blood should be taken at least 6 hours after a dose

**22 A**
Cancer patients receiving chemotherapy may be prescribed allopurinol as a prophylaxis for hyperuricaemia. See BNF, Chapter 10, section 2

23 D
See BNF, Chapter 2, section 4.1 under Thiazides and related diuretics under Cautions, further information. In hepatic failure, hypokalaemia caused by diuretics can precipitate encephalopathy

24 F
See BNF, Chapter 2, section 4.1 under Hepatic impairment. There is an increased risk of hypomagnesaemia in alcoholic cirrhosis

25 C
See BNF, Appendix 1, Interactions. Ciclosporin enhances the risk of hyperkalaemia, especially in patients with renal dysfunction

26 H
See BNF, Chapter 4, section 2.3 under Interactions. Lithium toxicity is made worse by sodium depletion; also, concurrent use of diuretics (particularly thiazides) is hazardous and should be avoided

27 A
Otomycosis (also known as Singapore ear) is a superficial mycotic infection of the outer ear canal caused by *Aspergillus niger*. It is more common in tropical countries and after prolonged treatment with antibiotics. See *Community Pharmacy*, 3rd edn (Rutter P; Churchill Livingstone, 2013)

28 G
See *Community Pharmacy*, 3rd edn (Rutter P; Churchill Livingstone, 2013)

29 B
*Chlamydia psittaci* may affect domestic bird owners and is an occupational disease of zoo and pet shop workers, poultry farmers and vets. Characteristic symptoms include splenomegaly, and should prompt consideration of this diagnosis if found in conjunction with pneumonia. See http://www.ccohs.ca/oshanswers/diseases/psittacosis.html

30 D
Legionnaires' disease is a severe, potentially fatal, acute pneumonia acquired by droplet inhalation of water contaminated by the bacterium *Legionella pneumophila*. British Thoracic Society (BTS) guidelines recommend investigations for legionella infection for all patients with severe community-acquired pneumonia, for other patients with specific risk factors and for all patients with community-acquired pneumonia during outbreaks. Most people become infected when they inhale microscopic water droplets containing legionella bacteria. This might be the spray from a shower, tap or whirlpool, or water dispersed through the ventilation system in a large building. Outbreaks have been linked to a range of sources, including hot tubs and whirlpools on cruise ships, cooling towers in air-conditioning systems, swimming pools, physical therapy equipment, and water systems in hotels, hospitals and nursing homes

31 H
See BNF, Chapter 5, section 2, Antipseudomonal penicillins. *Pseudomonas aeruginosa* can cause hospital-acquired pneumonia. Piperacillin with tazobactam has activity against a wider range of Gram-negative organisms than ticarcillin with clavulanic acid, and it is more active against *Pseudomonas aeruginosa*

32 C
See BNF, Chapter 13, section 2.3, under Ivermectin

33 E
See BNF, Chapter 5, section 4, under Mebendazole

34 D
See BNF, Chapter 13, section 2.3. Malathion is an organophosphorus insecticide that is used as an alternative for the treatment of head lice. Resistance may be an issue with this medicine

35 A
See BNF, Chapter 13, section 2.3. Dimeticone is effective against head lice (*Pediculus humanus capitis*), and acts on the surface of the organism by coating the head lice and interfering with water balance. This prevents the excretion of water by head lice and leads to rupture. It is less active against eggs and treatment should be repeated after 7 days

36 G
See BNF, Chapter 13, section 8. Pityriasis (tinea) versicolor can be treated with selenium sulfide shampoo (unlicensed indication). It can be used as a lotion (diluting with a small amount of water can reduce irritation) and left on the affected area for 10 minutes before rinsing off; it should be applied once daily for 7 days, and the course repeated if necessary

37 F
See BNF, Chapter 5, section 4. Praziquantel and pyrantel embonate (*Drontal*) may be used to deworm cats and are sold in pharmacies. It is effective against *Toxocara cati*, *Toxascaris leonina*, *Dipylidium caninum* and *Taenia taeniaeformis*. See http://www.noahcompendium.co.uk/Bayer_plc/Drontal_Cat_Tablets/-23595.html

38 A
See BNF, Chapter 13, section 2.2. Apply to infected nails once or twice weekly after filing and cleansing; allow to dry (approximately 3 minutes); treat fingernails for 6 months, toenails for 9–12 months (review at intervals of 3 months); avoid nail varnish or artificial nails during treatment. See RPS Amorolfine guidance at http://www.rpharms.com/support-resources-a-z/amorolfine-nail-lacquer-quick-reference-guide.asp

39 F
See BNF, Chapter 13, section 12. Silver nitrate may cause chemical burns on surrounding skin; it stains skin and fabric. Instructions in proprietary packs generally incorporate advice to remove dead skin before use by gentle filing and to cover with an adhesive dressing after application. *Bazuka* is known to irritate surrounding skin and damage fabric. It is the term burn and the staining properties of silver that fully define this answer

40 H
See BNF, Chapter 12, section 2.3. In hospital or in care establishments, mupirocin nasal ointment should be reserved for the eradication (in both patients and staff) of nasal carriage of meticillin-resistant *Staphylococcus aureus* (MRSA). The ointment should be applied three times daily for 5 days and a sample taken 2 days after treatment to confirm eradication

## SECTION D

1 D
See BNF, Chapter 2, section 8

2 F
See BNF, Chapter 2, section 1

3 E
See BNF, Chapter 2, section 4

4 B
See BNF, Chapter 2, section 6 (Hyperlipidaemia) under the monograph for simvastatin. There is a known interaction between simvastatin and amiodarone (which is used for treating atrial fibrillation). The simvastatin dose will need to be reduced to 20 mg OD to minimise this risk. Note that amlodipine is a distractor in this question as it is not used in atrial fibrillation

5 F
See responsible pharmacist legislation in relation to record keeping for 5 years

6 A
Patients with active treatment for cancer or cancer-related side-effects are exempt from prescription charges

7 A
Pregnant women are exempt from prescription charges

8 A
Inpatients in a hospital do not have to pay for their treatment

9 C
See MEP guide. CD register records need to be kept for 2 years from the last entry

10 C
See BNF, Appendix 3

11 F
See BNF, Appendix 3

12 B
See BNF, Appendix 3

13 E
See BNF, Appendix 3 and the side-effect profile of this drug

14 E
See BNF, Chapter 4, section 6

15 C
See BNF, Chapter 4, section 6. The MHRA/CHM released advice on this topic area in November 2013

16 F
Apply your general knowledge and controlled drugs legislation to this question

17 A
See BNF, Medical emergencies in the community

18 F
See BNF, Chapter 2, section 7.1

19 D
Some nitro-vasodilator products are available for OTC purchase

20 B
See BNF, Chapter 2, section 6 and section 7.1. The former states that statins are the drug of first choice for primary and secondary prevention

21 G
Black triangle drugs are intensively monitored

22 E
Flushing with calcium-channel blockers can be remedied by a dose reduction by the GP

23 F
Reactions to vaccinations must be reported even if they are not black triangle drugs

24 A
See BNF, Chapter 4, section 4, as well as MHRA/CHM advice released in August 2013 for more insight

25 C
See BNF, Chapter 4, section 4

26 E
See BNF, Chapter 1, section 8

27 G
See BNF, Chapter 4, section 5.2. Note that there are two choices, either:
(1) 300 mg OD for 1 day, increasing to 300 mg BD on day 2, and 300 mg TDS on day 3
OR
(2) 300 mg TDS, increased in steps of 300 mg every 2–3 days.
For this question the latter dosing applies based on the most suitable answer option

28 H
See BNF, section 6.2.2

29 A
See a good OTC or responding to symptoms textbook

30 B
Sertraline carries an increased risk of bleeding when given alongside NSAIDs; in this instance paracetamol as first choice is a reasonable suggestion

31 F
SSRIs can cause hyponatraemia

32 E
Long-term use of PPIs over 3 months to 1 year can lead to hypomagnesaemia

33 B
Pamidronate is used in cases of severe hypercalcaemia

34 F
See BNFC, Chapter 3, section 1. You will need to look at a suitable drug in step 3 of the BTS/SIGN guidance for a child aged 5–18 years

35 D
See BNFC, Chapter 3, section 1, under Severe acute asthma

36 G
This patient is on step 5 of the BTS/SIGN asthma guidance and so needs to have oral steroids next

37 C
See BNF, Chapter 6, section 3.3

38 B
See BNF, Chapter 6, section 3.1

39 A
See BNF, Chapter 6, section 3.3

40 H
See BNF, Chapter 6, section 3.1

# Calculation answers

**SECTION A**

1 57 mL
Need 26 mmol calcium ($Ca^{2+}$), therefore need 26 mmol of the calcium chloride hydrate ($CaCl_2{\cdot}2H_2O$)
Convert the molecular mass of this directly from g/mol to mg/mmol, thus 147.01 mg/mmol
Utilise and rearrange molar equation:

moles = mass ÷ molar mass → mass = moles × molar mass

Thus, mass of $CaCl_2{\cdot}2H_2O$ needed is 26 mmol × 147.01 mmol/mg = 3822.26 mg
13.4% = 13.4 g in 100 mL, thus 134 mg/mL
Therefore, 3822.26 mg ÷ 134 mg/mL = 28.52 mL
Note: two bags needed for the regimen (see top right of prescription), so 57.05 mL in total

2 5 ampoules
Same method as for Question 1
41.5 × 74.55 = 3093.825 mg KCl then 3093.825 mg ÷ 150 mg/mL = 20.6255 mL
Again, need enough for two bags so 41.251 mL in total from 5 ampoules

3 43.5 mL/hour
Divide the total volume of the bag (1044 mL) by the number of hours per bag (24 hours) to get 43.5 mL/hour

ANSWERS

4 37 mL/kg per day
Divide the total volume of the bag received in one day (1044 mL) by the patient's weight (28.6 kg) to get 36.5035 mL/kg per day. Remember to round up in this instance

5 16.7 mL
Use alligation method here:

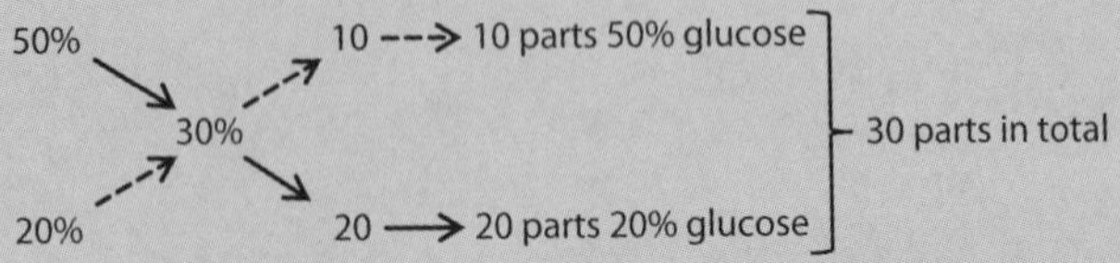


Need to make up 50 mL so 50 mL ÷ 30 parts = 1.6667 mL/part
Therefore, 1.6667 ml/part × 10 parts = 16.667 mL of the 50% glucose

6 8 mg/24-hour patch
From her immediate release she gets 50 × 4 = 200 mg dopamine
From her modified release she gets 1 × 100 × 0.7 = 70 mg dopamine
Thus, adjusted LEDD = 270 × 0.55 = 148.5 mg
Therefore, 148.5 ÷ 20 = 7.425 mg

7 410 mg
Even though this patient is slightly heavier than his ideal body weight (82 vs 79.9 kg), his actual body weight should be used because he is muscular, not obese
Therefore, loading dose = 5 mg/kg × 82 kg = 410 mg

8 377 mg
Because this patient is already taking aminophylline she does not require a loading dose, so the maintenance dose should be used here

IBW = 45.5 + (2.3 × 3) = 52.4 kg

She is elderly, so her dose = 0.3 mg/kg per hour × 52.4 kg = 15.72 mg per hour × 24 hours = 377.28 mg/24 hours

**9** 36.4 mL/hour
Can use the actual body weight of 52 kg here (see question 8)
She smokes so dose = 0.7 mg/kg per hour × 52 kg = 36.4 mg/hour
The infusion is 500 mg in 500 mL, thus 1 mg/mL
Therefore, 36.4 mL/hour needed

**10** 28.3 mL/minute
Candidates should know the Cockcroft–Gault formula and be able to utilise this in day-to-day care:

$$\text{CrCl} = [F \times (140 - \text{Age}) \times \text{Weight}] \div \text{SeCr}$$
$$= [1.23 \times (140 - 83) \times 54] \div 134 = 28.2538 \text{ mL/minute}$$

Note: $F$ is the correction factor for sex; male = 1.23, female = 1.04

**11** 98 tablets
The SPC states: 'The starting dose is 120 mg twice a day. After 7 days, the dose is increased to the recommended dose of 240 mg twice a day.'
Therefore, amount needed = (1 × 2 × 7) + (2 × 2 × 21) = 14 + 84 = 98 tablets

**12** Two bottles
Taking 5 mL QDS, thus 20 mL per day, and therefore 140 mL over the course of the week. This patient can be supplied both bottles as the course length is not longer than the expiry date on the made-up suspension

**13** 5.70 L/hour
First need to calculate IBW = 45.5 + (2.3 × 4) = 54.7 kg
Calculate CrCl using IBW = [1.04 × (140 − 67) × 54.7] ÷ 84 = 49.438 mL/minute
Therefore, DigCl = (0.06 × 49.438) + (0.05 × 54.7) = 5.70128 L/hour

**14** 250 mcg
IBW = 50.0 + (2.3 × 12) = 77.6 kg, therefore need to use actual body weight
CrCl = [1.23 × (140 − 74) × 75] ÷ 153 = 39.7941 mL/minute
DigCl = (0.053 × 39.7941) + (0.02 × 75) = 3.6091 L/hour
Need to rearrange $C_{pss}$ equation to find $D$. Also, $F$ becomes 0.63 (due to 63% bioavailability)
Therefore, $D = [C_{pss} \times (\text{DigCl} \times t)] \div F = [2.0 \times (3.6091 \times 24)] \div 0.63 = 274.9782$ mcg

ANSWERS

15 66%
This is a percentage difference calculation
Therefore, percentage predicted $FEV_1 = (1.39 \div 2.10) \times 100 = 66.1905\%$

16 25 g
Dose needed is 0.8 g/kg × 28 kg = 22.4 g
Therefore, two 10-g vials and one 5-g vial should be supplied

17 11 hours and 26 minutes
Concentration of *Intratect* is 10 g/200 mL = 1 g/20 mL
Thus, volume of *Intratect* is 22.4 g × 20 mL/g = 448 mL
Rate of infusion is 1.4 mL/kg per hour × 28 kg = 39.2 mL/hour
Therefore, 448 mL ÷ 39.2 mL/hour = 11.4286 hours = 11 hours and 25.71 minutes

18 8 hours and 41 minutes
Need to calculate the volume infused at every rate increase:

1.4 mL/kg/hour for 30 minutes = (1.4 × 28) × 0.5 = 19.6 mL
1.5 mL/kg/hour for 15 minutes = (1.5 × 28) × 0.25 = 10.5 mL
1.6 mL/kg/hour for 15 minutes = (1.6 × 28) × 0.25 = 11.2 mL
1.7 mL/kg/hour for 15 minutes = (1.7 × 28) × 0.25 = 11.9 mL
1.8 mL/kg/hour for 15 minutes = (1.8 × 28) × 0.25 = 12.6 mL

Total volume = 65.8 ml in 1.5 hours
Volume left to infuse at 1.9 mL/kg/hour= 448 − 65.8 = 382.2 mL
Rate of infusion is 1.9 × 28 = 53.2 mL/hour
Thus, 382.2 mL ÷ 53.2 mL/hour = 7.1842 hours
Therefore, total time = 7.1842 + 1.5 = 8.6842 hours = 8 hours and 41.052 minutes

19 15.95 g
Total mass that needs to be made is 16 g (16 suppositories)
Displacement by morphine = 16 × 5 mg ÷ 1.6 = 50 mg
Therefore, mass of base (witepsol) = 16 000 mg − 50 mg = 15 950 mg = 15.95 g

20 3.30 g
10% excess of 150 g = 150 × 1.1 = 165 g
Formula states 20 g salicylic acid in 1000 g ointment, thus 0.02 g in 1 g
Therefore, 0.02 × 165 = 3.3 g

ANSWERS

**21** 1.62 $m^2$
BSA = $[(130 \times 73) \div 3600]^{0.5} = 2.6361111^{0.5} = 1.62361\ m^2$

**22** 78.8 mcg
$125 \times 0.63 = 78.75$ mcg

**23** 7.0 mL/hour
Dose per minute = $3 \times 62 = 186$ mcg/minute $\times$ 60 minutes = 11 160 mcg/hour = 11.16 mg/hour
Bag contains 160 g in 100 mL = 1.6 mg/mL
Therefore, 11.16 mg/hour $\div$ 1.6 mg/mL = 6.975 mL/hour

**24** 22.5 mL
Find equivalent syrup dose: $150 \times 0.9 = 135$ mg
30 mg/5 mL = 6 mg/mL
Therefore, 135 mg $\div$ 6 mg/mL = 22.5 mL

**25** 280 ampoules
Each flucloxacillin 1-g vial requires two 10-mL water for injection ampoules
Thus, drug requirements = $(2 \times 2) \times 4 \times 14 = 224$ ampoules
Do not reuse sterile WFI ampoules, so each flush needs one 10-mL WFI ampoule
Thus, flush requirements = $1 \times 4 \times 14 = 56$ ampoules
Therefore, total number of ampoules needed = 224 + 56 = 280 ampoules

**26** 246 mg
Dose = $15 \times 16.4 = 246$ mg

**27** 0.7 mL
Note: the question states regular dose so need to work with 15 mg/kg, not 20 mg/kg (STAT dose)
Dose = $15 \times 1.14 = 17.1$ mg per dose
Suspension = 120 mg/5 mL = 24 mg/mL
Therefore, volume per dose = 17.1 mg $\div$ 24 mg/mL = 0.7125 mL

**28** 4 mL
Dexamethasone contains 3.3 mg/mL of injection
Therefore, volume = 13.2 mg $\div$ 3.3 mg/mL = 4 mL

29 40 mL
The maximum concentration allowed is 600 mg in 10 mL = 60 mg/mL
The dose prescribed is 2400 mg
Therefore, volume needed = 2400 mg ÷ 60 mg/mL = 40 mL

30 303.0 mg
Alligation should be used here:

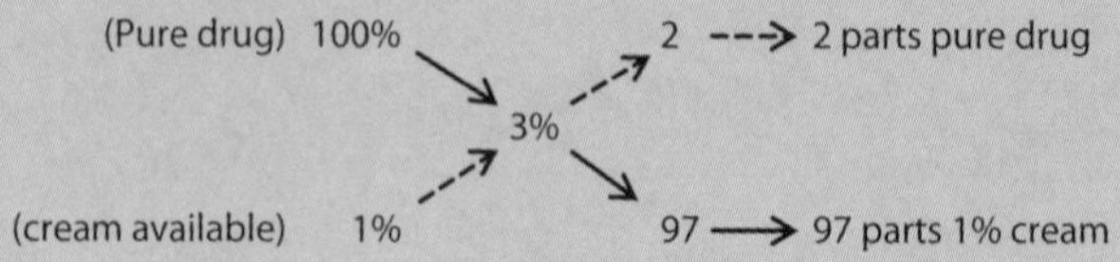


Thus, the 1% cream makes 97 parts of final 99 parts: 15 g/99 = 0.151515 g/part
Therefore, 2 parts × 0.151515 g/part = 0.30303 = 303.03 mg zinc oxide to add
Can check answer: ([150 + 303.03]/[15000 + 303.03]) × 100 = 2.9603%



31 20 mg/mL
Final concentration = 0.05% = 0.05 g in 100 mL = 0.0005 g/mL = 0.5 mg/mL
Amount of chlorhexidine in 200 mL solution is 0.5 × 200 = 100 mg
This 100 mg came from the 5 mL of the original solution
Therefore, 100 mg in 5 mL = 20 mg/mL

32 60.76 mg/10 mL
Allocate the values for the equation:

$f = 0.577$ (remove the minus, as the cerebrospinal fluid freezing point depression causes it to freeze at −0.577°C)
$a = 0.227$ (the value given is for 1% solution, therefore 2 × 0.1135 = 0.227)
$b = 0.576$

Putting these into the equation gives you $W = 0.60764\%$ (g/100 mL)
Therefore, 0.060764 g/10 mL = 60.764 mg/10 mL

33 1.97

Only one $pK_a$ given so assume $[H^+]$ is same as $[A^-]$, therefore $K_a = [H^+]^2 \div [HA]$

$[HA]$ = molar concentration of drug, thus in 1 L = 15 g $L^{-1}$ ÷ 138.21 g·$mol^{-1}$ = 0.1085 M

Convert $pK_a$ to $K_a$ so: $10^{-pKa} = 10^{-2.97} = 1.07152 \times 10^{-3}$

Rearrange $K_a$ equation so $[H^+]^2 = K_a \times [HA]$

Thus $[H^+] = \sqrt{}(K_a \times [HA])$

Therefore, $[H^+] = \sqrt{}(1.07152 \times 10^{-3} \times 0.1085) = 0.01078$

Finally, pH = $-\log [H^+] = -\log 0.01078 = 1.967$

34 3 vials

Number of vials = (72 × 3.23) ÷ 100 = 2.3256

35 60 mL

See SPC, section 4.2

Iron dose (mg) = body weight (kg) × {[target haemoglobin (g/dL) – actual haemoglobin (g/dL)] × 2.4} + depot iron (mg)

Thus, dose = 54 × {[14 – 8.6] × 2.4} + 500 = 1199.84 mg

Therefore, volume required (mL) = iron dose (mg) ÷ 20 mg/mL = 59.992 mL

36 51.9%

Run time is the same, so can just use the number of tablets per minute

Thus, (4100 ÷ 2700) × 100 = 151.85%; therefore, a 51.85% increase

Test: (2700 × 0.5185) + 2700 = 4099.95

37 30 mg

Candidates should know that the usual breakthrough pain dose is one-sixth to one-tenth of the total daily morphine equivalent dose. See prescribing in palliative care information at the start of the BNF

Total daily dose = 90 + 90 = 180 mg

Thus, one-sixth of this = 180/6 = 30 mg

38 32.7 kg

BMI ($kg/m^2$) = Weight (kg) ÷ [Height (m) × Height (m)]

Candidates should be able to derive this equation from the question if they cannot remember it

Rearrange to find weight: $W = BMI \times H^2$

Thus, target weight = $24 \times 1.67^2 = 66.9336$ kg

Therefore, weight needed to be lost = 99.6 – 66.9339 = 32.6664 kg

ANSWERS

39 86.9 mmol
Sodium bicarbonate dissociates into equal concentrations of sodium and bicarbonate ions
Thus, the bag delivers 150 mmol/L × 0.5 L = 75 mmol to the patient
The patient is getting 5.95 × 2 = 11.9 mmol sodium from the tablets
Therefore, total sodium given = 11.9 + 75 = 86.9 mmol

40 2 mL
Half a tablet gives 5 mg hydrocortisone so the dispersion contains 5 mg/10 mL = 0.5 mg/mL
Therefore, 2 mL needed for morning dose and 1 mL for the next two doses

## SECTION B

1 20.0 mL
BNF dose = 4 mg/kg BD Weight of child = 4.7 kg
$4 \times 4.7 = 18.8$ mg
$18.8 \times 2 = 37.6$ mg
$37.6 \times 5 = 188$ mg
188 mg of 50 mg/5 mL
100 mg/10 mL
10 mg/1 mL
1 mg/0.1 mL
188 mg/18.8 mL
Dispense 20 mL and advise patient to discard after 5 days

2 1.9 mL
1 mg/0.1 mL = 18.8 mg/1.88 mL
Dose = 1.9 mL BD for 5 days

3 378 tablets
ONE in the morning for 2 weeks: $1 \times 14 = 14$
ONE in the morning and ONE in the evening for 2 weeks: $(1 + 1) \times 14 = 28$
TWO in the morning and ONE in the evening for 2 weeks: $(2 + 1) \times 14 = 42$
TWO in the morning and TWO in the evening for 2 weeks: $(2 + 2) \times 14 = 56$
THREE in the morning and TWO in the evening for 2 weeks: $(3 + 2) \times 14 = 70$
THREE in the morning and THREE in the evening for 4 weeks: $(3 + 3) \times 28 = 168$
TOTAL: $14 + 28 + 42 + 56 + 70 + 168 = 378$ tablets

4 13.8 mL
$C1 \times V1 = C2 \times V2 = 10 \times V1 = 0.5 \times 276$, so $V1 = 138/10 = 13.8$ mL
OR
2 mL in 40 mL = 0.5 mL in 10 mL = 0.05 mL in 1 mL = 276 mL $\times$ 0.05 = 13.8 mL
OR
(276 mL/40 mL) $\times$ 2 mL = 13.8 mL

5 1.82 L
26% v/v = 26 mL/100 mL = 260 mL/L = 260 mL/L $\times$ 7 = 1820 mL/7 L

ANSWERS

6 92.6 mL
C1 × V1 = C2 × V2 = 68 × V1 = 0.09 × 70 000 = V1 = 0.09 × 70 000/68 = 92.6 mL
OR alternatively:
0.09% w/v = 0.09 g/100 mL
In 70 L we have (0.09 × 10 × 70) = 63 g
We have a 68% w/v concentrate; we need to find what volume contains 63 g of Drug A
68 g/100 mL, therefore (63)/(68/100) = 92.6 mL

7 23.7
BMI = Weight (kg)/Height $(m)^2$ = 1.59 × 1.59 = 2.53 = 60/2.53 = 23.7

8 7.32 g
200 mg chloral hydrate in 5 mL = 400 mg in 10 mL = 400 mg/10 mL = 40 mg/1 mL = 40 × 183 = 7320 mg
OR alternatively:
200 mg chloral hydrate in 5 mL of preparation
Hence 40 mg chloral hydrate in 1 mL of preparation
Therefore (40 × 183) mg in 183 mL of preparation
= 7320 mg = 7.32 g



9 20.58 g
7 × 300 mg = 2100 mg or 2.1 g amount of zinc oxide needed for 7 suppositories
5 g of zinc oxide displaces 1 g of the base. 1 g displaces 0.2 g of the base
2.1 g × 0.2 = 0.42 g amount of cocoa butter displaced by 2.1 g of zinc oxide
3 g × 7 = 21 g amount of cocoa butter needed for unmedicated suppositories
0.42 g of the base will be displaced by zinc oxide so, 21 g – 0.42 g = 20.58 g

10 4.62 mL/minute
Dose: 30 mg/kg over 5 minutes
For a 77-kg patient = 30 × 77 = 2310 mg over 5 minutes = 462 mg/minute
*Epilim* IV = 400 mg in 4 mL = 100 mg in 1 mL, so 462 mg = 4.62 mL
Therefore, injection rate = 4.62 mL/minute

**11** 8.4 mL
25 × 5.6 = 140 mg every 8 hours
TDD = 420 mg
*Augmentin* 600 mg or co-amoxiclav 500/100 = 500 mg amoxicillin in 10 mL = 50 mg/mL
420/50 = 8.4 mL

**12** 2.88% w/w
360 g 5% w/w = 360 × 5/100 = 18 g
275 g 1% w/w = 275 × 1/100 = 2.75 g
18 g + 2.75 g = 20.75 g total amount of calamine
360 g + 275 g + 85 g WSP = 720 g
(20.75 g/720 g) × 100 g = 2.88% w/w

**13** 0.125 mg
1 in 40 000 = 1 g in 40 000 mL = 1000 mg in 40 000 mL = 1 mg in 40 mL = 1000 mcg in 40 mL = 125 mcg in 5 mL = 0.125 mg/5 mL

**14** 150 mg
0.5% = 500 mg/100 g = 5 mg/1 g
5 mg × 30 = 150 mg weight in 30 g

**15** 131.25 mg
In one week patient will use 1050 mL of a 1 in 8000 solution
Pharmacist to make solution 20 times this strength = 1 in 400
Therefore, the pharmacist needs to make 52.5 mL of 1 in 400
1 in 400 = 1 g in 400 mL = 0.25 g/100 mL = 250 mg/100 mL = 25 mg/10 mL = 125 mg/50 mL = 6.25 mg/2.5 mL = 131.25 mg/52.5 mL

**16** 124 tablets
5 days 40 mg = 8 tablets = 8 × 5 = 40 tablets
3 days 35 mg = 7 tablets = 7 × 3 = 21 tablets
3 days 30 mg = 6 tablets = 6 × 3 = 18 tablets
3 days 25 mg = 5 tablets = 5 × 3 = 15 tablets
3 days 20 mg = 4 tablets = 4 × 3 = 12 tablets
3 days 15 mg = 3 tablets = 3 × 3 = 9 tablets
3 days 10 mg = 2 tablets = 2 × 3 = 6 tablets
3 days 5 mg = 1 tablet = 1 × 3 = 3 tablets
Total 40 + 21 + 18 + 15 + 12 + 9 + 6 + 3 = 124 tablets for the course

OR alternatively:
$(8 \times 5) + ([1 + 2 + 3 + 4 + 5 + 6 + 7]) \times 3)$
$(8 \times 5) + (28 \times 3) = 124$ mL

17 156 drops
Day 1: 4 times/hour × 6 = 24 drops
Day 1: 2 times/hour × 18 = 36 drops
Day 2: 1 time/hour = 24 drops
Days 3–14 = 6 times/24 hours = 6 × 12 days = 72 drops = 24 + 36 + 24 + 72 = 156 drops

18 2 bottles
20 drops/1 mL = 100 drops/5 mL of *Ciloxan* = 2 bottles needed

19 4 g
$C_1M_1 = C_2M_2 = 0.05 \times M_1 = 0.02 \times 10 = 0.05 \times M_1 = 0.2 = M_1 = 0.2/0.05 = 4$ g

20 10 mL TDS
Child's dose = 1200/100 × 25 = 300 mg = given TDS,
so at each dose = 300/3 = 100 mg
Solution = 50 mg/5 mL = 10 mg/mL; so, for 100 mg,
need 100/10 = 10 mL

## SECTION C

1 9.75 mg
2.5 mcg × 65 kg × 60 minutes = 9750 mcg = 9.75 mg

2 105 tablets
150 mg ON for 5 days = 30 tablets
125 mg ON for 5 days = 25 tablets
100 mg ON for 5 days = 20 tablets
75 mg ON for 5 days = 15 tablets
50 mg ON for 5 days = 10 tablets
25 mg ON for 5 days = 5 tablets
Total = 105 tablets

3 20 mL
12 mg × 6.6 kg = 79.2 mg per day
V = 2 mg/1 mL
79.2/$x$ mL
$x$ = 39.6 in two doses = 19.8 = 20 mL

4 0.25 mL
Total morphine dose = 180 × 2 = 360 mg daily
According to table, equivalent to 120 mg diamorphine
120 mg/24 = 5 mg every hour
20 mg in 1 mL
5 mg in $x$ mL
$x$ = 0.25 mL required every hour

5 7 mL to 11.5 mL
One-tenth to one-sixth of total daily dose (140 mg)
14 mg to 23 mg every 2–4 hours
7 mL to 11.5 mL every 2–4 hours PRN

6 490 mL
The syrup is 10 mg/5 mL
Week 1: 15 mg ON → 7.5 mL × 7 = 52.5 mL
Week 2: 25 mg ON → 12.5 × 7 = 87.5 mL
Weeks 3–4: 25 mg BD → 12.5 × 2 × 14 = 350 mL
Total = 490 mL

7 6 mL
500 mcg × 6 kg = 3000 mcg = 3 mg
1 mg = 1000 mcg
62.5 mg/125 mL
3 mg/$x$ mL
$x$ = (125 × 3) /62.5 = 6 mL

8 1.8 $m^2$
1.5 m = 150 cm
BSA = (150 cm × 80)/3600 = $3.33^{0.5}$ = 1.8 $m^2$

9 30 tablets
1.5 × 40 × 5 = 300/10 = 30 tablets

10 42.5 hours

| Hours | Plasma concentration (mcg/mL) |
|---|---|
| 0 | 74 |
| 8.5 | 37 |
| 17 | 18.5 |
| 25.5 | 9.25 |
| 34 | 4.625 |
| 42.5 | 2.3125 |

At 42.5 hours the plasma concentration will reach 2.3125 mcg/mL

11 100 mcg
1 g in 10 000 mL= 100 mcg

12 11 hours and 20 minutes
2 L/1 minute
1360 L/$x$ minutes
$x$ = 680
680/60 = 11.33
11 hours and 20 minutes

13 15 units
Apomorphine injection = 20 mg/2 mL
Dose = 1.5 mg → (1.5/20) × 2 = 0.15 mL

Each syringe can hold 100 units/1 mL
i.e. 10 units/0.1 mL
and 15 units in 0.15 mL

**14** 50 g
0.25% w/v = 0.25 g in 100 mL
0.125 g in 50 mL
0.125 g must be in 2.5 mL
1000/2.5 = 400
400 × 0.125 = 50 g

**15** 6 hours 40 minutes
10 g in 100 mL
25 g in 250 mL
25 g/minute
1000/25 = 400

**16** 225 mg
150 mg/36 mm/24 hours increased to: 54 mm/24 hours
= (150 mg × 54 mm)/36 mm = 225 mg

**17** 32 mL
According the BNF: 'Rifampicin 600 mg every 12 hours for 2 days; child under 1 year 5 mg/kg every 12 hours for 2 days; 1–12 years 10 mg/kg every 12 hours for 2 days.'
10 mg × 16 kg = 160 mg every 12 hours
100 mg/5 mL
160 mg/$x$ mL; $x$ = 8 mL
8 × 2 = 16 mL per day × 2 days = 32 mL

**18** 4.9 g
2.8 g in 100 g; 2.8 + 2.1 = 4.9 g

**19** 9.4 % w/v
20 g + 10 g + 7.5 g = 37.5 g
37.5/400 = 0.09375 = 9.4% w/v

20 315 tablets

| | | | |
|---|---|---|---|
| 10 tablets | 7 days | 70 | |
| 9 tablets | 7 days | 63 | |
| 8 tablets | 7 days | 56 | |
| 7 tablets | 7 days | 49 | |
| 6 tablets | 7 days | 42 | |
| 5 tablets | 7 days | 35 | = 315 tablets |

## SECTION D

1 50 mL
Using the alligation method you will find that 20 parts of the 50% injection and 20 parts of the 10% infusion are needed to make the 30% solution. This equates to 50 mL of each (when making a 100 mL solution)

2 17.56 mL/minute per 1.73 $m^2$
Using the equation provided and knowing that 1 foot is equivalent to 30 cm:

$(40 \times 180)/410$
$= 7200/410$
$= 17.56$

3 5 mL
1 in 20 dilution, therefore, for 100 mL we need 5 mL of concentrated chloroform water

4 10 mL
This changeover is a straight dose-for-dose switch as both products contain phenytoin base
Therefore, 60 mg = 10 mL of the 30 mg/5 mL suspension

5 2.5 g
$C_1M_1 = C_2M_2 \rightarrow 1\ M_1 = 0.025 \times 100$
$1\ M_1 = 2.5$

6 168 units
Dose = 0.5 mg/kg BD = 12 units BD
For a 1-week period, this amounts to 12 × 2 × 7 units = 168

7 147 tablets
$60 \times 0.8 = 48$ mg (round to 50 mg)
$40 \times 0.8 = 32$ mg (round to 30 mg)
$20 \times 0.8 = 16$ mg (round to 15 mg)
$10 \times 0.8 = 8$ mg (round to 10 mg)
Total = $(10 + 6 + 3 + 2) \times 7$
Total = $21 \times 7 = 147$

ANSWERS

**8** 50 mL
1 mL TDS = 3 mL/day
$(3 \times 14) + 8 = 50$ mL

**9** 250 mL
$C_1V_1 = C_2V_2 \rightarrow 50\ V_1 = 25 \times 500$
$50\ V_1 = 12\,500$
$V_1 = 1250/5 = 250$ mL

**10** 500 mg
0.1% = 0.1 g in 100 g
Therefore, 0.5 g in 500 g
$0.5 \times 1000 = 500$ mg

**11** 7.5 seconds
$2.5 \times 60 = 150$ mg
$150/20 = 7.5$



**12** 0.01 %
1 in 10 000 mL = 0.1 in 1000 mL = 0.01 in 100 mL = 0.01%

**13** 9.2 mmol
$2.3 \times 4 = 9.2$ mmol

**14** 60 000 units
150 000/30 = 5000 units/drop
$5000 \times 12 = 60\,000$

**15** 10 mmol
Total potassium required for neonate $\rightarrow 3 \times 2 = 6$ mmol
Total fluid volume/day $\rightarrow 150 \times 2 = 300$ mL
Therefore, 6 mmol potassium in 300 mL
We need to create a 500 mL solution, therefore need to upscale quantities:
$500/300 \times 6 = 9.99$ mmol (= 10 mmol for practicality)

**16** 500 mg
1 g in 1000 mL, therefore 500 mg in 500 mL

**17** 432 mg
10 mcg/kg per minute; weight = 60 kg
$10 \times 60 \times 60 = 36\,000$ mcg/h, i.e. 36 mg/hour
$36 \times 12 = 432$ mg

**18** 125 mg/L
If initial plasma level is 1 g/L, then after 6 hours it will be 500 mg/L, after 12 hours it will be 250 mg/L and after 18 hours it will be 125 mg/L

**19** 54 mL
From extract provided, 3 mL/kg of glucose 5% is required as a diluent; child's weight = 18 kg
$3 \times 18 = 54$ mL

**20** 13 mL
Dose = $250 \times 1.3\ \text{m}^2 = 325$ mg
$325/25 = 13$ mL

**21** 30 mg/L
Initial amount is 40 mg on ingestion, at 6 hours it is 20 mg, therefore at 12 hours it will be 10 mg
$40 - 10 = 30$ mg/L eliminated

**22** 2.25 mmol
Calcium gluconate contains 225 micromol/mL
Therefore, in 10 mL we have 2250 micromol, i.e. 2.25 mmol

**23** 20 mg
1 g in 1000 mL, therefore 20 mg in 20 mL

**24** 53 mg
Patient is having a total daily oral morphine dose of $(60 \times 2) + (10 \times 4) = 160$ mg
Morphine to subcutaneous diamorphine is a one-third reduction
$1/3 \times 160 = 53$ mg
Note: for this question we have utilised the subcutaneous infusions section (under 'prescribing in palliative care' in the BNF and not the 'equivalent doses of opioid analgesics' table (which specifies a 10-mg dose of oral morphine is equivalent to a 3-mg dose of diamorphine)

25 14.4 g
12.5 g/100 g, therefore 14.375 g/115 g (14.4 to one decimal place)

26 4 g
The trick with this question is to work backwards from the final concentration
1 in 500 = 1 g/500 mL, i.e. 50 mL of original solution = 1 g
We have 200 mL of original solution, therefore 4 g
You can then re-check this: we have a 4 g solution (in 200 mL), we take 50 mL (1 g) and dilute this to 500 mL, i.e. we now have a 1 in 500 (or 1 g in 500 mL) solution

27 280 mg
$(1.5 \times 0.56)/3 = 0.28$ g (i.e. 280 mg)

28 15 vials
$0.4 \times 72.45 = 28.98$ g – this is rounded to 30 g
$30 \times 5 = 150$ g over 5 days
$150/10 = 15$ vials

29 20 mL
A 1:1 dilution is required to go from 8.4% to 4.2%, i.e. 20 mL of 8.4% + 20 mL of water for injection will give a 4.2% concentration

30 432 mg
$8/100 \times 400 = 32$
$400 + 32 = 432$ mg
Alternatively, $(108/100) \times 400 = 432$ mg

# Index